EMERGENCIES

Edited by: Ibrahim M. Eltorai, MD and James K. Schmitt, MD
Foreword by: Joel A. DeLisa, MD, MS

in Chronic Spinal Cord Injury Patients

3RD EDITION

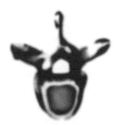

Preface to First Edition

Emergencies in Chronic Spinal Cord Injury Patients is a volume of articles presented in a seminar held at the VAMC in Long Beach, California on June 1, 1984.

The editor felt that there was a great need for such a seminar for the practitioners faced with a patient with chronic spinal cord injury (SCI) presenting with an emergency condition.

There is no doubt that SCIs will continue to occur. And with the improvement in acute care and rehabilitation programs from all aspects, there will be more chronic patients seen, particularly because the longevity of these patients has tremendously increased. While striving to develop a cure for the so far "incurable" injury, it is very important to deal with the emergencies in the chronic patient. SCI has tremendous repercussion on bodily functions below the level of injury. There is a tremendous psychological impact due to a complete change in lifestyle. Even the pharmacokinetics in these individuals is different post-injury. Drug metabolism and disposition has been shown to be substantially changed by the injury and only recently has valid criteria for drug administration been discovered to aid the practitioner in a rational approach to drug therapy in SCI.

It appears that even the medical profession has little understanding of the magnitude of the problems related to SCI. For these reasons, the Long Beach seminar has been put into this volume. It is not intended to be a detailed, comprehensive textbook, but an adequate reference for the busy practitioner. Each contributor describes a plan for managing the peculiar emergency condition that may be encountered. This is largely based on the author's personal experience.

The editor hopes that the seminar's material on this important subject will help practitioners deal with emergencies in the chronic spinal cord injured.

Ibrahim M. Eltorai, MD Editor

Preface to Second Edition

The first edition of this manual entitled *Emergencies in Chronic Spinal Cord Injury Patients* and published in 1988 was welcomed by many emergency room physicians and nurses. It is intended to be a quick reference for general practitioners involved in the care of patients with spinal cord injury (SCI) as well as general practitioners who encounter these patients occasionally. The format of the first edition has been retained as it has proven useful to house officers on duty. All sections have been updated and new sections have been added.

This reference is dedicated to all the contributors who kindly worked hard on their manuscripts with their only compensation being better quality assurance for the care of patients with SCI. The book is also dedicated to Eastern Paralyzed Veterans Association without whose generosity it would not have existed.

The book is not intended to be encyclopedic and adequate reference with each chapter can be of help for further reading. The authors are among the most experienced in the field of SCI and they take all the responsibility for their contributions. The authors and the editor join in anticipation that this book will meet an urgent need by the emergency physicians, nurses, students, and allied health professionals who treat patients with SCI.

Ibrahim M. Eltorai, MD Editor

Preface to Third Edition

This text was written and published twice in the last 10 years. It was written primarily for the practitioners giving care to patients with spinal cord injury (SCI) as well as to the caregivers not familiar with the subject. The purpose was to develop guidelines for management of emergencies in patients with chronic SCI. It is our experience over the years that unoriented medical staff may not realize the differences in pathophysiology of SCI. We will give a few examples:

I. A patient with autonomic dysreflexia may be diagnosed as essential hypertension not realizing that the hypertension is a result of a plugged catheter or impacted rectum and the patient may develop a cerebrovascular accident.

II. A patient with bowel perforation may be misdiagnosed as having fecal impaction (constipation) and may be operated on late with high mortality and morbidity. However, a patient with adynamic ileus secondary to spinal cord inhibitory reflexes was operated on for an acute abdomen with negative findings.

III. A patient with a fracture was put in a circular cast and developed gangrene.

IV. A patient with septic arthritis of the hip secondary to a pressure sore was scheduled for hip disarticulation. He could have been treated with an upper femorectomy and plastic reconstruction, thus saving the limb.

V. In another example, patients having occlusive arterial disease of lower extremity have been scheduled for amputation, but the limbs were salvaged by an angioplasty and medical treatment with adjunctive hyperbaric 02 therapy.

Many other examples could be mentioned. That is why this text has been written. The faculty has been selected among the most experienced in the field of spinal cord impairment. The text is not an encyclopedia but it offers important avenues for consultation. Sufficient references are also available.

Ibrahim M. Eltorai, MD Editor

James K. Schmitt, MD Co-Editor

Contributors

Brent A. Armstrong, MD Assistant Professor of Medicine, Staff Physician, General Internal Medicine, VA Medical Center, Richmond, VA 23249.

Anousheh Behnegar, MD Department of Rehabilitation Medicine, Mount Sinai School of Medicine, New York, NY 10029.

Helen T. Bosshart, ACSW/LCSW SCI Home Care Coordinator, VA Medical Center, Augusta, GA 30904-6285.

Thomas C. Cesario, MD Professor of Medicine, Dean of University of California, College of Medicine, Irvine, CA 92697.

Robert Conroy, MD Associate Professor, University of California, Irvine, CA; Chief of Interventional Radiology, VA Medical Center, Long Beach, CA 90822.

Anita Cordova, MSN, CRRN VA Long Beach Healthcare System, Long Beach, CA 90808.

Ibrahim M. Eltorai, MD Assistant Clinical Professor of Surgery, University of California, Irvine Medical Center, Orange, CA; Senior Surgeon, SCI Service, VA Medical Center, Long Beach, CA 90822.

T. Scott Gallacher, MD, MS Fellow, Pulmonary and Critical Care Section, University of California (Irvine), Irvine, CA; VA Medical Center, Long Beach, CA 90822.

Douglas Garland, MD Clinical Professor, Department of Orthopedics, University of Southern California, Los Angeles, CA; Chief of Neurotrauma, Surgery Department, Rancho Los Amigos National Rehabilitation Center, Downey, CA 90242.

Regina M. Hovey, MD Assistant Clinical Professor of Surgery, Division of Urology, University of California Irvine Medical Center; Chief of Urology SCI Service, VA Medical Center, Long Beach, CA 90822.

Diane L. Huntington, RRT Registered Respiratory Therapist in Charge of Respiratory Care, SCI Service, VA Medical Center, Long Beach, CA 90822.

James G. Jakowatz, MD Associate Professor of Surgery and Surgical Oncology, University of California, College of Medicine, Irvine, CA; Staff Surgeon, VA Medical Center, Long Beach, CA 90822.

George L. Juler, MD Emeritus, Adjunct Professor of Surgery, University of California, College of Medicine, Irvine, CA; Consultant Surgeon, VA Medical Center, Long Beach, CA 90822.

Robert A. Kaplan, MD Assistant Clinical Professor of Medicine, University of California College of Medicine, Irvine Medical Center, Orange, CA; Staff Physician, Medical Service, VA Medical Center, Long Beach, CA 90808.

Bok Y. Lee, MD, FACS Professor of Surgery, New York Medical College, Valhalla, NY; Director of Surgical Research, Sound Shore Medical Center, New Rochelle, NY; Adjunct Professor of Bioengineering, Rensselaer Polytechnic Institute, Troy, NY.

Kenneth G. Lehmann, MD Associate Professor of Medicine, University of Washington School of Medicine, Seattle, WA; Chief, Cardiac Catheterization Laboratory, VA Puget Sound Health Care System, Seattle, WA 98108.

C. Kees Mahutte, MD, PhD Professor of Medicine, University of California (College of Medicine), Irvine, CA; Chief Pulmonary and Critical Care Section, VA Medical Center, Long Beach, CA 90822.

Norma D. McKenzie, MD Associate Professor of Psychiatry, Virginia Commonwealth University, Medical College of Virginia, Richmond, VA.

Meena Midha, MD Associate Professor of Physical Medicine and Rehabilitation, Chief, SCI Service, VA Medical Center, Richmond, VA 23249.

Robert E. Montroy, MD Clinical Associate Professor of Surgery, University of California College of Medicine, Irvine Medical Center, Orange, CA; Chief, Plastic Surgery Section of the Surgical Service; Assistant Chief, SCI Service, VA Medical Center, Long Beach, CA 90822.

Shireesha Narla, MD SCI Service, VA Medical Center, Richmond, VA 23249.

James N. Nelson, MD Chief Psychiatry Consultant, SCI Service, VA Medical Center, Long Beach, CA 90822.

Bernard A. Nemchausky, MD, FACP Chief, Spinal Cord Impairment/Dysfunction, Attending in Gastroenterology, Associate Professor in Medicine, Loyola University, Stritch School of Medicine; Chief, SCI Service, VA Medical Center, Hines, IL 60141.

Cathy Parsa, BSN, MA, CRRN Program Coordinator, Comprehensive Rehabilitation Health Care Group, VA Medical Center, Long Beach, CA 90822.

R. Kannan Rajan, MD Clinical Associate Professor of Medicine, University of California College of Medicine, Irvine, CA; Staff Physician Department of Medicine and SCI Service, VA Medical Center, Long Beach, CA 90822.

James K. Schmitt, MD Professor of Medicine, Chief General Internal Medicine, Associate Chief of Medicine, VA Medical Center, Richmond, VA 23249.

Leslie Shokes, MD Spinal Cord Injury Service, Rancho Los Amigos National Medical Center, Downey, CA 90242.

Marcalee Sipski, MD Chief of SCI Service, Associate Professor of Clinical Neurologic Surgery, VA Medical Center, Miami, FL 33125.

Rodney M. Wishnow, MD Associate Professor of Medicine and Microbiology, University of California, College of Medicine, Irvine, CA; Staff Physician, VA Medical Center, Long Beach, CA 90822.

Robert M. Woolsey, MD Professor of Neurology, St. Louis University School of Medicine, St. Louis, MO; Chief, SCI Service, VA Medical Center, St. Louis, MO 63125.

Dedication

This text is dedicated to Mr. James J. Peters,

Executive Director of Eastern Paralyzed Veterans Association, in recognition of his superb efforts for betterment of the care and saving lives of the individuals with spinal cord impairments, and for devoting his time gracefully and unselfishly to these patients.

"The actions of men are the best interpreters of their thoughts."

In Memoriam

The Editors are grateful to Angela Wu, Director of Library Services, Eastern Paralyzed Veterans Assocation, for her tremendous efforts in preparing this book. Without her dedication and efficiency, this book would not have been published. Her contributions in the field of SCI will be deeply missed.

Acknowledgments

It should be obvious that this text could not have been written without the encouragement of Eastern Paralyzed Veterans Association (EPVA), headed by its Executive Director, Mr. James J. Peters, who gave carte blanche to write this edition. We would like to express our deep gratitude to Mr. Peters. Special thanks go to Ms. Angela Wu, MLS, Director of EPVA Library and Information Services. Without her help in organizing the manuscripts and managing this project, nothing could have materialized. Our thanks cannot be enough for the contributors who did an excellent job in spite of their heavy schedules. We hope that this text will help spinal cord injury care providers in emergency situations, especially when they are faced by an acute problem for the first time. Our intention was to simplify the topics; more details can be found in the references or in other sources of literature.

Ibrahim M. Eltorai, MD Editor

James K. Schmitt, MD Co-Editor

Foreword

Individuals with chronic spinal cord injury (SCI) present a host of challenges to the clinicians who care for them. The typical signs and symptoms of many disorders are often lacking, requiring us to maintain a high level of suspicion for those that threaten further disability or even death. The profound physiologic changes associated with SCI also require us to reevaluate traditional therapeutic modalities in this setting. Because of the stresses of living with chronic disability, and dependency on a complex network of support, we must be prepared to handle psychosocial as well as psychiatric emergencies, which can have serious long-term consequences for people with SCI. Care by SCI nursing specialists can help minimize emergencies through early intervention and by instituting care plans aimed at preventing complications.

This third edition of *Emergencies in Chronic Spinal Cord Injury Patients* addresses many of these wide-ranging issues. This updated guide provides a practical approach to the types of emergencies likely to be encountered in the population with SCI. Each chapter, authored by experts in the field, addresses a specific aspect of emergency management. This text is essential for clinicians who have limited experience with patients with SCI. Specialists in spinal cord medicine will find a useful review of the state-of-the-art of emergency management.

Joel A. DeLisa, MD, MS
|Editor, *The Journal of Spinal Cord Medicine*
|Professor and Chair, Department of PM&R, UMDNJ—
New Jersey Medical School
|President and CEO, Kessler Medical Rehabilitation Research
and Educational Corporation

Table of Contents

AUTONOMIC DYSREFLEXIA

James K. Schmitt, MD; Meena Midha, MD;
Norma D. McKenzie, MD; Shireesha Narla, MD

CHAPTER ONE

Of all the emergencies that befall the patient with spinal cord injury (SCI), autonomic dysreflexia is the emergency that comes the closest to being unique to patients with SCI. Patients who have undergone injuries to the brainstem, such as tumor resection and brain trauma, also may experience autonomic dysreflexia, but the mechanism is similar to that in the patient with SCI.[1] Knowledge of the diagnosis and treatment of autonomic dysreflexia is important for clinicians caring for these patients because it is preventable, readily treatable, and if untreated, may lead to death.[2] Furthermore, autonomic dysreflexia may be a sign of other serious medical conditions, such as an acute abdomen.[3]

Mechanism of Autonomic Dysreflexia [1,4,5]

The sympathetic division of the autonomic nervous system has its cells of origin in the preganglionic cell bodies located in the interomediolateral gray columns of the spinal cord from T1 through L2. The preganglionic fibers terminate in the paravertebral ganglia that give rise to postganglionic sympathetic fibers. The postganglionic fibers innervate the heart, arteries, and veins. Activation of these neurons results in increase in blood pressure and pulse. SCIs above T6, therefore, result in hypotension and a tendency toward bradycardia in the unstimulated state. (Rarely lesions as low as T8 may cause autonomic dysreflexia.)

|In normal subjects, loud noises or cutaneous stimuli increase blood pressure and heart rate secondary to central activation of the sympathetic nervous system. In patients with tetraplegia, interruption of descending sympathetic pathways prevents these effects. In ambulatory subjects, stimuli, such as a distended viscus or cutaneous stimuli, would tend to raise the blood pressure by activation of the splanchnic bed via the sympathetic nervous system. However, this reflex is inhibited by sympathetic activity that originates above T6. Furthermore, any increase in blood pressure will stimulate baroreceptors in the carotid sinus and in the aorta, which in turn send impulses to the vasomotor center of the brain via the ninth and tenth cranial nerves. Efferent impulses from the vasomotor center through the tenth nerve result in slowing of the heart and inhibition of sympathetic outflow leading to vasodilation and a fall in blood pressure.

|In the patient with high SCI, however, inhibition of the sympathetic reflex is blocked by the SCI. The vagus nerve is not injured by SCI and the increase in blood pressure results in a reflex slowing of the heart, which is not sufficient to cause an adequate fall in blood pressure. Therefore, SCIs above T6 result in relatively unopposed sympathetic outflow following a variety of stimuli.

|Norepinephrine and 5-hydroxytryptamine normally suppress anterior horn cell activity. Biochemical studies have found that following SCI there is an accumulation of norepinephrine and 5-hydroxytryptamine above the lesion, but these substances disappear below the lesion.[1] Gamma amino benzoic acid, which is an interneuronal inhibitor, decreases as well. Substance P, which may initiate synaptic events, increases below the cord lesion. It is postulated that substance P and other neurotransmitters, uninhibited by norepinephrine and 5-hydroxytryptamine, set the biochemical stage for autonomic dysreflexia.

|A stimulus such as bladder distension results in the afferent impulse traveling up the cord and stimulating the sympathetic chain. These impulses are blocked at the level of the cord lesion. As a result, hypertension, tachycardia, and other adrenergic manifestations including piloerection and skin pallor may occur below the level of the cord lesion. Activation of the parasympathetic nervous system results in slowing of the heart, sweating and flushing above the level of the cord lesion, mydriasis, conjunctival congestion, and Horner's syndrome. Reflex vasodilation occurs only above the cord lesion.

|It is possible that the observed effects on blood pressure and pulse are due in part to upregulation of sympathetic receptors due to decreased sympathetic activity in the basal state.[1] Studies using microneurographic tracings of muscle sympathetic nerves during bladder stimulation indicate that there is rapid activation of the sympathetic nervous system. Plasma norepinephrine levels rise immediately, peak with the blood pressure response and correlate with the magnitude of the blood pressure rise.[6] Plasma epinephrine levels fail to rise, indicating that the adrenal gland does not play a part in autonomic dysreflexia.

|From the above considerations it is clear the higher and more complete the cord lesion, the more severe the episode of autonomic dysreflexia will be. Some causes of autonomic dysreflexia are listed in Table I.

Table I **Some Causes of Autonomic Dysreflexia** [7]

I.	Bladder distension
II.	Fecal impaction
III.	Acute abdomen
IV.	Sexual intercourse
V.	Deep vein thrombosis
VI.	Pulmonary emboli
VII.	Reflex sympathetic dystrophy [8]
VIII.	Heterotopic bone formation
IX.	Invasive procedures
X.	Pain
XI.	Pressure sores
XII.	Medications [9]
XIII.	Labor and delivery [10]
XIV.	Functional electrical stimulation [11]
XV.	Fractures, dislocations, and other traumas

Diagnosis of Autonomic Dysreflexia [1,4,5]

|The first episode of autonomic dysreflexia may occur any time from a few months to many years after the period of spinal shock. The most common symptom of autonomic dysreflexia is headache. The complaint of a new headache in a patient with SCI should always result in a determination of the blood pressure. The systolic blood pressure in a patient with tetraplegia or high paraplegia ranges from 90 to 100 mm Hg, so a blood pressure of 130 systolic in such an individual may represent an elevation. Other symptoms of autonomic dysreflexia not described above include blurred vision or spots in the patient's visual fields, nasal congestion, apprehension, cardiac arrhythmias including atrial fibrillation, and premature ventricular contractions. The triad of headache, sweating, and cutaneous vasodilation is almost diagnostic of autonomic dysreflexia. Uncommonly, the first manifestation of autonomic dysreflexia is a seizure.[12]

|Autonomic dysreflexia resembles pheochromocytoma in its presentation.[13] However, the clinical characteristics of these disorders differ (Table II). Furthermore, whereas autonomic dysreflexia is common in patients with SCI with a reported prevalence as high as 66% to 85%, in individuals with tetraplegia pheochromocytoma is rare, occurring in fewer than 1 per 1,000 of hypertensive patients.

|Not all cases of autonomic dysreflexia are symptomatic. In some instances, the only manifestation is increased blood pressure following a stimulus, such as voiding.[14]

Table II Clinical Characteristics of Autonomic Dysreflexia and Pheochromocytoma

	Autonomic dysreflexia	Pheochromocytoma
Hypertension	present intermittently	present (may be intermittent)
Headache	often present	occasionally
Provoked by visceral stimuli	usually	rarely
Vasodilation above cord level	present	absent
Sweating	localized to upper body or unilateral	diffuse
Bradycardia during paroxysm	often	absent
Unilateral Horner's syndrome	occasionally present	absent
Urinary catecholamines	normal	elevated

Modified from Schmitt J, Adler R. Endocrine metabolic consequences of spinal cord injury. Phys Med Rehab 1987;1:436.

Treatment of Autonomic Dysreflexia [1, 7, 15]

|Bringing a patient from supine to upright may immediately reduce the blood pressure. Clothing and constrictive devices should be loosened. The etiology of the autonomic dysreflexia should be searched for because rapid relief of the cause may reverse the dysreflexia faster than medication. Because bladder obstruction is the most common cause, this is the first area that should be investigated, unless another cause is obvious. If there is an indwelling catheter, kinks in the tubing should be removed. If this fails to restore urine flow, the catheter should be gently irrigated with normal saline at body temperature following instillation of 2% lidocaine gel, which blocks efferent impulses. Stimuli, such as tapping on the bladder or manually compressing it, should be avoided. If irrigation fails to relieve the problem, the catheter may be replaced, again instilling viscous lidocaine prior to inserting the catheter. If a catheter is not in place, one should be inserted to check for urinary retention.

|If investigation of the bladder fails to reveal the cause of autonomic dysreflexia, a fecal impaction should be sought. Viscous lidocaine should be instilled into the rectum first. If a fecal impaction is discovered, an attempt should be made to disimpact it. If removal of bladder or rectal obstruction results in a normalization of blood pressure, the blood pressure should be monitored for two hours. Other rapidly treatable causes, such as contact with sharp objects, should be sought.

|If the above measures fail to normalize the blood pressure, medication should be started. It has not been established what level of blood pressure constitutes an immediate risk to the patient. The Consortium for Spinal Cord Medicine has established a blood pressure of 150 mm Hg systolic as the level at which pharmacological therapy should be instituted.[7] From the known mechanism of autonomic dysreflexia, the most effective drugs are those that modify sympathetic tone.[15] Vasoactive drugs or adrenolytic agents are therefore the drugs of choice. Immediate-acting nifedipine is perhaps the most commonly used agent. The most effective mode of delivery is bite and swallow. (Sublingual nifedipine is absorbed erratically.) Alternately, 1 inch of 2% nitroglycerine paste may be applied to the skin above the level of SCI. If hypotension occurs, the paste may be quickly wiped off. Other medications that may be used are alpha-adrenergic blockers (such as phenoxybenzamine or prazosin) or direct-acting vasodilators such as hydralazine, nitroprusside, or intravenous nitroglycerine (Table III). The blood pressure and pulse should be determined every 2 to 5 minutes until the patient is stable.

Table III **Some Pharmacological Treatments of Autonomic Dysreflexia**

Drug	Dose and Interval
Nifedipine*	10 mg P.O. (may repeat after 30 minutes if necessary)
Nitroglycerine Ointment 2%	1 inch to upper chest or back (additional inch may be given after 15 minutes if needed)
Nitroprusside	0.5 to 1.5 mg/min IV
Hydralazine	25 to 100 mg P.O. or 20 to 40 mg IV or IM
Labetalol	20 mg IV (may repeat every 10 minutes with doses of 20 to 80 mg to maximum dose of 300 mg)
Diazoxide	Bolus of 50 to 100 mg every 10 to 15 minutes or infusion of 15-30 mg/min
Phenoxybenzamine	10 mg P.O. twice daily (higher doses up to 60 mg/day may be required)
Prazosin	2.5 mg P.O. twice daily

*Editor's note: Because of adverse outcomes with sublingual nifedipine, some experts have recommended against the use of this drug. However, it's still a commonly used agent.

|If the cause of autonomic dysreflexia is unclear or the hypertension fails to respond to upright posture and oral medication, the patient should be hospitalized. When parenteral agents are used the patient should be in an intensive care unit. Nitroprusside and nitroglycerine (5–100 micrograms/min) drips have the advantage of being rapidly reversible with discontinuation of therapy. Beta blockers, by allowing unopposed alpha-tone, may increase the blood pressure in hyperadrenergic states, such as pheochromocytoma. From these considerations pure beta blockers should probably be avoided in the treatment of the hypertension of autonomic dysreflexia. If the patient becomes hypotensive on medication he or she should be returned to the supine position.

|After the episode of autonomic dysreflexia has been reversed (blood pressure and pulse restored to normal and there are no other symptoms), it should be discussed in the patient's medical record describing the presenting symptoms, pulse, blood pressure, and response to treatment.

Prevention of Autonomic Dysreflexia

|In many instances, autonomic dysreflexia can be prevented.[1, 7, 16] Avoidance of bladder distension by intermittent catheterization can prevent the hypertensive crisis. Likewise, prevention of or early treatment of fecal impaction may prevent autonomic dysreflexia. Some authorities recommend that patients with high cord injuries have a diagnostic cystometrogram to determine the likelihood of developing autonomic dysreflexia.[17] Early diagnosis of gastrointestinal emergencies such as appendicitis, prevention of deep vein thrombosis, early treatment of infection, and pain may prevent autonomic dysreflexia.

|Bladder training and self-catheterization will prevent autonomic dysreflexia by preventing distension. In some situations, performance of transurethral sphincterectomy will be necessary in order to prevent bladder distension and avoiding an indwelling catheter. In situations that are high risk for the production of autonomic dysreflexia, such as cystoscopy or electroejaculation, medication may be given prophylactically. Use of xylocaine gel in the urethra prior to cystoscopy or in the rectum prior to the rectal exam may prevent autonomic dysreflexia.

|In a situation in which the patient is at particularly high risk of autonomic dysreflexia, nifedipine 10 mg P.O. may be given 30 minutes prior to the procedure and repeated as necessary. Nifedipine given twice daily is effective in the prophylaxis of autonomic dysreflexia.[18] The patient and the family should be taught the precipitating factors and signs and symptoms of autonomic dysreflexia.

Conclusion

|Autonomic dysreflexia is a common emergency in patients with SCI with lesions at T6 and above. Stimuli, such as bladder distension and fecal impaction, result in activation of sympathetic spinal reflexes that cause vasoconstriction and hypertension below the cord level and vasodilation above the level of the lesion. The most common symptoms of autonomic dysreflexia are headache, upper body sweating, and visual symptoms.

|The immediate treatment of autonomic dysreflexia consists of raising the patient to the upright position and searching for a correctable cause. The most common medications used are nifedipine 10 mg and nitroglycerine ointment.

References

1. Lee B, Karmaker M, Herz B, et al. Autonomic dysreflexia revisited. *J Spinal Cord Med* 1995;18:75-87.

2. Eltorai I, Kim R, Vulpe M, et al. Fatal cerebral hemorrhage due to autonomic dysreflexia in a tetraplegic patient: case report and review. *Paraplegia* 1992;30:355-360.

3. Longo W, Vernava A. The Neurogenic Bowel In: Young R, Woolsey R (eds). *Diagnosis and Management of Disorders of the Spinal Cord.* WB Saunders: Philadelphia, 1995, pp. 331-344.

4. Arrowood S, Mohanty P, Thames M. Cardiovascular problems in the spinal cord injured patient. *Phys Med Rehabil: State Art Reviews* 1987;1:443-445.

5. Colachis S. Autonomic hyperreflexia with spinal cord injury. *J Am Paraplegia Soc* 1992;15:171-186.

6. Mathias C, Christensen N, Corbett J, et al. Plasma catecholamines during paroxysmal neurogenic hypertension in quadriplegic man. *Circ Res* 1976;39:204-208.

7. *Acute Management of Autonomic Dysreflexia.* Clinical Practice Guidelines. 1997; Paralyzed Veterans of America.

8. Clinchot D, Colachis S. Autonomic hyperreflexia associated with exacerbation of reflex sympathetic dystrophy. *Spinal Cord Med* 1996;19:255-257.

9. Wineinger M, Basford J. Autonomic dysreflexia due to medication: misadventure in the use of isometheptene combination to treat migraine. *Arch Phys Med Rehabil* 1985;66:645-646.

10. McGregor JA, Meeuwsen J. Autonomic hyperreflexia: a mortal danger for spinal cord-damaged women in labor. *Am J Obstet Gynecol* 1985;151 (3):330-333.

11. Ashley E, Laskin J, Olenik L, et al. Evidence of autonomic dysreflexia during functional electrical stimulation in individuals with spinal cord injuries. *Paraplegia* 1993;31:593-605.

12. Yarkony G, Katz R, Wu Y. Seizures secondary to autonomic dysreflexia. *Arch Phys Med Rehabil* 1986;67:834-835.

13. Schmitt J, Adler R. Endocrine metabolic consequences of spinal cord injury. *Phys Med Rehabil: State Art Reviews* 1987;1:425-441.

14. Linsenmeyer T, Campagnolo D, Chou I. Silent autonomic dysreflexia during voiding in men with spinal cord injuries. *J Urol* 1996;155:519-522.

15. Segal J. Clinical pharmacology of spinal cord injury. In: Young R, Woolsey R. (eds) *Diagnosis and Management of Disorders of the Spinal Cord.* WB Saunders: Philadelphia, 1995, pp. 414-438.

16. Thyberg M, Ertzgaard P, Gylling M, et al. Effect of nifedipine on cystometry-induced elevation of blood pressure in patients with a reflex urinary bladder after a high level spinal cord injury. *Paraplegia* 1994;32:308-313.

17. Trop C, Bennett C. Autonomic dysreflexia and its urological implications: a review. *J Urol* 1991;146:146-149.

18. Lindam R, Leffler E, Kedia K. A comparison of the efficacy of an alpha 1 adrenergic blocker and a slow calcium channel blocker in the control of autonomic dysreflexia. *Paraplegia* 1985;23:34-38.

Acute and Chronic | Kenneth G. Lehmann, MD

|CARDIOVASCULAR PROBLEMS

CHAPTER TWO ▃▃▃▃▃▃▃▃▃▃▃▃

|Great strides have been made in the care of spinal cord injuries (SCI) since Harvey Cushing's report of an 80% mortality rate during World War I.[1] However, only in recent years have antibiotic therapy, assisted ventilation, urologic treatment, and general rehabilitative care been able to offer hope for prolonged survival in patients with high-level SCI. Historically, SCI programs have been directed toward the care and needs of the acutely injured rather than the patients with chronic SCI, and program goals have been focused on the resolution of problems accompanying immediate, post-acute rehabilitative processes.[2] Research efforts as well have concentrated upon this critical but relatively short period.[3]

|However, the demographics are changing. The young continue to represent the majority of new spinal injuries, with 70% of fresh injuries occurring between the ages of 17 and 35.[4] Excluding the immediate post-injury period, life expectancy in SCI now approaches that of the general population.[4] This increased survival is reflected in the shifting age distribution cared for by the VA Health System, with more than 60% of all veterans with SCI now over the age of 45 years.[5] In addition, death from infection and renal insufficiency is beginning to give way to diseases of modern Western man, with cardiovascular ailments predominating. Wide and unpredictable fluctuations in arterial pressure and heart rate that commonly occur in high level SCI can be troublesome in the young, but could prove life threatening in the aged individual.

|Over the past years, it has been observed that cardiovascular emergencies occurring in patients with SCI are sometimes not handled appropriately or expeditiously. There are several reasons for this failure to provide optimal care. First, many physicians unfamiliar with SCI approach these individuals with fear or ignorance of their altered cardiovascular physiology. A prime example of this phenomenon is that of autonomic dysreflexia. A lack of awareness of this syndrome is common, and has led to disastrous circumstances on occasion. For example, an individual with quadriplegia died during a barium enema because treatment for his dysreflexic episode was directed only at the reflex bradycardia, without recognition of the severe hypertension that inevitably occurs. Second, patients with chronic SCI often manifest symptoms that differ from classic presentations of cardiovascular diseases. Third, frequently there is a failure to differentiate expected cardiovascular perturbations that are transient and self-limiting from true cardiac emergencies requiring immediate attention. Fourth, there is a conspicuous lack of careful scientific investigation and rigorous data pertaining to cardiovascular alterations in SCI. Without these data, clinicians are left with only anecdotes and educated guesses by which to guide their therapeutic approach. This inexcusable gap in knowledge needs to be corrected before definitive advice on the handling of cardiovascular emergencies can be formulated.

Alterations in Cardiovascular Physiology

High level vs. low level injury: The response of a patient with chronic SCI to cardiovascular diseases and emergencies is greatly affected by the level of SCI. Patients with paraplegia with injuries in the low thoracic or lumbar cord possess nearly intact autonomic innervation to their heart and vasculature. Hence, their responses to both the underlying cardiovascular disease process as well as to pharmacologic intervention are generally similar to the responses shown by individuals without SCI. Conversely, people with quadriplegia with injuries to the cervical or high thoracic cord lose all or nearly all sympathetic control throughout the cardiovascular system. Parasympathetic influences, due to their exit from the central nervous system at the level of the brain stem, remain intact. This "central sympathectomy" can have a profound influence on cardiovascular unction, with the autonomic imbalance that results greatly affecting the sympathetic/parasympathetic equilibrium that represents the cornerstone of the autonomic nervous system. Several clinically important manifestations of this state have been observed. We have shown that severe acute injury to the cervical spinal cord in man is regularly accompanied by alterations in cardiovascular function, including bradyarrhythmias, asystole, marked hypotension, supraventricular tachyarrhythmias, and atrioventricular block.[6-8] In addition, these individuals experience a statistically significant increase in primary cardiac arrest, often proving fatal. These abnormalities were not found in patients with injuries of the thoracic or lumbar cord. Patients with chronic high-level SCI exhibit an enhanced pressor response to norepinephrine infusion.[9-10] Although this was initially thought to be a manifestation of Cannon's law of denervation hypersensitivity,[9] several features distinguish SCI from other related disorders of autonomic function, including its preganglionic lesion. We have found a heightened chronotropic response to isoproterenol infusions, even when blood pressure is maintained at its basal level to eliminate the contribution to altered baroreflex influence. This hyperresponsiveness should be kept in mind when administering any sympathomimetic agent to chronic patients with quadriplegia.

Completeness of injury: Because of its influence on autonomic function, the completeness of cord injury can obviously have a substantial effect on cardiovascular emergencies and their treatment. It is difficult *a priori* to predict responses in a given individual with partial injury due to the variability of neurologic impairment. It is frequently impossible using historical data or patient interview to determine the completeness of injury. We have found that the cold pressor test, using ice immersion of the hand (or ice pack applied to the forehead, if hand sensitivity is diminished) is useful for documenting the presence of central sympathetic dysfunction in patients with partial high level injury.

Duration of injury: In patients with quadriplegia, the duration of injury can play a major role in the patient's response to cardiovascular perturbations or pharmacologic intervention. In a study of 71 patients with acute severe injury to the spinal cord (admitted within 12 hours of trauma), we found a high prevalence of marked bradycardia, significant hypotension, and cardiac arrest in patients with severe cervical, as opposed to thoracolumbar, injuries.[6] See Table I below.

Table I **Comparison of Effects of Spinal Injuries**

Clinical Results	Severe Cervical (n = 31)	Milder Cervical (n = 17)	Thoracolumbar (n = 23)	
persistent bradycardia	31 (100%)	6 (35%)	3 (13%)	⁕
marked bradycardia	22 (71%)	2 (12%)	1 (4%)	⁕
atropine/pacer therapy	9 (29%)	0	0	⁕⁕
hypotension	21 (68%)	0	0	⁕
pressor therapy	11 (35%)	0	0	⁕⁕
primary cardiac arrest	5 (16%)	0	0	⁕⁕⁕
Electrocardiographic Results				
repolarization changes	7 (32%)	4 (29%)	5 (33%)	
corrected QT (mean ± *SD*)	.432 ± 043	.424 ± 043	.416 ± 038	
new AV block	4 (18%)	0	0	⁕⁕⁕
supraventricular tachycardia	6 (19%)	1 (6%)	0	
ventricular tachycardia	2 (6%)	0	0	

⁕ overall $p < 0.00001$, Group 1 vs Group 2 $p < 0.001$, Group 1 vs Group 3 $p < 0.0001$. ⁕⁕ overall $p < 0.001$, Group 1 vs Group 2 $p < 0.02$, Group 1 vs Group 3 $p < 0.01$ ⁕⁕⁕ overall $p < 0.05$

|Interestingly, these cardiovascular disturbances in all instances resolved spontaneously 2-6 weeks after injury. Although this adaptive response is obviously beneficial, the chronic stage of cervical SCI is marked by its own set of cardiovascular abnormalities. Chief among these is autonomic dysreflexia.[11] This condition, common to most people with quadriplegia, is characterized by transient episodes of profound hypertension, diaphoresis, reflex bradycardia, and piloerection, along with flushing above and vasoconstriction below the level of injury.[12,14] To date, the mechanism of this apparent mass sympathetic reflex has not been established, and no fully satisfactory treatment has been discovered. The details of this important and fascinating phenomenon are described elsewhere in this book.

Acute Myocardial Infarction

Predisposing factors: With most patients with SCI now living to their sixth, seventh, and eighth decades, coronary artery disease is becoming an increasingly recognized problem. Patients with SCI also appear to be more predisposed to this condition, in part because of the relative inactivity of most of these patients, as well as the episodic hypertension that often accompanies chronic high level SCI. It is important to address modifiable risk factors as early as possible, including control of hypertension and hypercholesterolemia, cessation of smoking, adequate exercise (when possible), diagnosis and tight control of diabetes, and maintenance of ideal body weight.

Clinical presentation: Acute myocardial infarction (MI) in a patient with SCI can present either with classic symptoms or with an unusual symptom complex that is difficult to categorize. The typical pressing, squeezing, band-like substernal chest pain may be present. However, in individuals with high-level injury, these symptoms may be significantly altered or missing altogether. Other potential symptoms include a vague sense of uneasiness, diaphoresis, gastrointestinal upset, and autonomic dysreflexia. With many episodes of acute MI undoubtedly "silent," the patient with SCI may present several days later with symptoms of fatigue, heart failure, or post-infarct angina. Therefore, it is important to maintain a high index of suspicion when patients with SCI present with complaints that could possibly be related to acute MI. Measurement of new markers of myocardial injury may be useful in this regard. In particular, troponin I and troponin T are both sensitive and specific, and can be used to diagnose a myocardial infarction occurring anywhere between 6 hours and 10 days after symptom onset.

Pseudo-infarct pattern: The diagnosis of acute MI is further complicated by recently recognized electrocardiogram(ECG) patterns in chronic patients with quadriplegia that can easily mimic acute infarction. We have shown that 65% of patients with chronic cervical SCI show baseline ST segment elevations in excess of 1 mm in multiple electrocardiographic leads (especially in V_2, V_3, and V_4).[14] This pattern was quite similar to that seen with "early repolarization variant" often found in young athletic individuals. Although this ST segment elevation did not respond to exercise, a low-dose isoproterenol infusion promptly restored ST height to normal, implicating an autonomic imbalance as the primary disturbance. Clinically, the only importance of this observation is its mimicry of other acute cardiac events, such as myocardial infarction and pericarditis. One helpful clue is that the ST segments associated with high-level SCI maintain their normal concave upward appearance. In contrast, the current of injury pattern associated with acute infarction usually appears convex upward.[14]

Pharmacologic management: In general, management of acute MI does not differ substantially between individuals with and without SCI. Patients presenting early in the course of infarction (generally, less than 12 hours) should be strongly considered for thrombolytic therapy with agents such as tissue plasminogen activatior(tPA) or streptokinase. Note that clear-cut ST segment elevation (or new left-bundle branch block) should be present in a pattern that is different from the pseudo-infarct pattern discussed above. Some individuals with SCI will have relative contraindications to the use of thrombolytics, including bleeding from indwelling catheters, but this should not dissuade the clinician from a careful assessment of risk/benefit because of the well-documented improvement in mortality and morbidity with the use of these drugs. Primary angioplasty with or without intracoronary stent placement represents a good alternative to thrombolytics in centers capable of this procedure, especially if contraindications to thrombolysis exist. It is clear that aspirin can cause a significant reduction in mortality during acute MI, with this effect additive to that seen with thrombolytic therapy. Therefore, one aspirin tablet should be chewed and swallowed immediately upon presentation. Intravenous nitroglycerin can be useful in reducing the pain associated with peri-infarct ischemia, and may help with long-term outcome as well. The use of this drug should be encouraged where appropriate, but due to its pre-load reducing effect, its dose should be slowly and closely titrated in the SCI population. The importance of adequate analgesia cannot be forgotten, with opiates such as morphine sulfate representing the drugs of choice for this condition. Other adjunctive therapies, such as supplemental oxygen, heparin, lidocaine for severe arrhythmias, and diuretics for pulmonary edema and/or heart failure, should be administered as indicated. Beta-blocking agents can be used, but only with caution, as they can manifest accentuated or paradoxical effects in this group of patients. The use of ultra-short-acting beta-blocking agents, such as esmolol, should be used first when possible.

Unstable Angina

Management: The management of unstable angina does not differ greatly between individuals with and those without SCI. Aspirin, intravenous nitroglycerin, unfractionated heparin, and analgesics all play important roles in this syndrome. Newer agents for the treatment of unstable angina include the platelet glycoprotein IIb/IIIa inhibitors (tirofiban, eptifibatide, and abciximab) and low-molecular-weight heparins (enoxaparin and dalteparin). Appropriate use of these newer drugs has reduced mortality and recurrent infarction by 10% to 30%, but all carry a significant risk of bleeding and should be prescribed and monitored by someone familiar with their use. The use of intraaortic balloon counter-pulsation may be limited by the small caliber of the femoral and iliac arteries often found in these individuals due to atrophy of the lower extremity musculature. Coronary angioplasty and coronary bypass surgery are viable options for patients with SCI, but only when undertaken by anesthesiologists, surgeons, and cardiologists who understand the nature and treatment of problems peculiar to SCI.

Diagnosis of coronary artery disease: Because of their inability to perform standard lower extremity exercise, the diagnosis of coronary artery disease (CAD) in patients with SCI with chest pain syndromes can be difficult. Fortunately, alternate forms of cardiovascular stress are available. Pharmacologic stress is widely employed in the diagnosis of CAD. Both dipyridamole (Persantine) and adenosine are used to produce potent coronary vasodilation and elicit relative imbalances of coronary blood flow. These are generally performed in conjunction with radionuclide scintigraphy. Of these two agents, the latter is probably preferable in the SCI population due to its very short half-life. Stress echocardiography appears as sensitive and specific as radionuclide scintigraphy, with the choice between these two techniques largely dependent on local expertise. Unfortunately, both of these tests are expensive and may not be readily available to all SCI practitioners. As an alternative, we have used arm ergometry extensively in this group of patients, and have found it to produce satisfactory results, albeit at a lower predicted workload than what occurs with standard treadmill exercise in normal individuals. Careful lead placement and attachment is critical to help reduce ECG motion artifact. An intermittent protocol (i.e., one with a 20-second pause between each stage) may be useful in permitting attainment of better ECG tracings and blood pressure measurement by arm sphygmomanometry. We have found that the hands of patients with quadriplegia can be successfully strapped to pedals of an ergometer using Ace wraps. Wheelchair ergometers are now commercially available, and may represent a better choice, as the physiologic stress more closely mimics that experienced in everyday life for the patient with SCI. Atrial pacing via an esophageal lead or transvenous atrial lead can produce graded and controlled increases in heart rate in patients unable to exercise. As with exercise testing, the ECG can be monitored for signs of ischemia (principally horizontal or downsloping ST-segment depression). Finally, cardiac catheterization and coronary angiography can always be used when needed for definitive diagnosis or to assess severity and candidacy for cardiac intervention.

Differentiating Chest Pain Syndromes

|It is important to recognize that not all chest pain originates from coronary artery disease. Two of the most important differential diagnoses of acute MI are aortic dissection and pulmonary embolism because of their life-threatening nature if not promptly recognized and treated. Both are also more likely to occur in the SCI population. Aortic dissection is more common in patients with severe hypertension and might be particularly anticipated in individuals with poorly controlled autonomic dysreflexia. Pulmonary embolism increases in likelihood with immobility and venostasis, conditions that are common to the SCI population. Hence, it is critical that the triad of acute MI, aortic dissection, and pulmonary embolism are immediately considered in the individual presenting with acute severe chest pain. Acute pericarditis may also present with chest pain that is classically pleuritic and positional in nature. As mentioned previously, the ECG of patients with complete high-level chronic SCI can often mimic acute pericarditis due to the diffuse ST segment elevations present in both conditions. Gastrointestinal symptoms, such as reflux, can also produce chest pain symptoms indistinguishable from angina. Finally, musculoskeletal diseases and fractures are common in SCI, and atypical characteristics may mimic other more serious causes of chest pain.

Bradyarrhythmias

Predisposition of high level injury: As stated previously, severe bradycardia and hypotension are common immediately after high-level SCI, presumably due to the acute withdrawal of sympathetic tone to the heart and vasculature. Over a 2- to 6-week period, these parameters trend back toward normal, although we and others have found relative bradycardia and hypotension as common features of chronic quadriplegia. Related forms of bradycardia may also be found, including bradycardia with a junctional escape rhythm, and various forms of atrioventricular block.

Importance of hemodynamic response: The importance of bradyarrhythmias lies largely in their accompanying hemodynamic alterations. Many athletes and patients with high-level SCI can run baseline heart rates in the 40s with no lightheadedness or other evidence of cerebral hypoperfusion. Hence, it is important not to use an absolute value of heart rate as the principal criterion for treatment. Chronic asymptomatic bradycardias often do not require treatment. On the other hand, intervention is usually required for symptomatic bradycardia, especially in the setting of another acute cardiovascular event.

Use of anticholinergic agents: As stated previously, the bradyarrhythmias in high-level SCI often result from the autonomic imbalance imposed upon the heart by intact parasympathetic (vagal) tone combined with absent sympathetic tone. Therefore, the reduction in vagal tone with the use of anticholinergic drugs can be useful. All individuals possess an "intrinsic" heart rate (typically in the range of 110 beats per minute) that reflects the activity of sino-atrial node in the absence of autonomic influences. In theory, it should be possible to accelerate the heart rate of most patients with high-level SCI up to that point using drugs such as atropine. High doses of the drug (up to 0.04 mg/kg) may be required to obtain the desired effect.

Use of sympathomimetic agents: By replacing deficient sympathetic tone, it may first appear sympathomimetic drugs should be the treatment of choice for sinus bradyarrhythmias. However, these agents may also lead to undesirable side effects, such as inappropriate arterial vasodilatation induced by interaction with ß_1 adrenoceptor binding without the competitive influence of an α- adrenoceptor response. These drugs should therefore be used with caution. Moreover, it is important to recognize the sympathetic hypersensitivity that regularly occurs in patients with high-level SCI. We have tried a number of agents for this problem, including isoproterenol, terbutaline, epinephrine, and ephedrine. Although none has proved ideal, we have found that very low-dose isoproterenol can sometimes be used to support low heart rates without excessively lowering arterial pressure. Oral ephedrine can be used as an alternative when intravenous medication cannot be given.

Use of temporary pacers: Temporary pacemakers represent an important alternative to drugs when the bradyarrhythmias are profound or sustained. Although the insertion of temporary pacing wires is commonly accomplished using the transvenous approach, this technique must be performed cautiously in individuals with SCI. I can clearly recall the necessity of bilateral chest tubes in a 24-year old patient with acute cervical SCI after multiple attempts at achieving central venous access for pacing by two competent cardiology fellows at Yale/New Haven Hospital. There are two principal reasons for this increased risk. First, many patients with acute and chronic SCI manifest low venous volume and tone. Therefore, cannulation of the central venous circulation can be difficult due to collapsed veins and poor return of blood flow. Second, the patients are often immobilized due to braces and/or there are practical difficulties in moving patients to standard fluoroscopy tables. Cutaneous transthoracic temporary pacemakers represent a logical alternative to the transvenous approach, and should be strongly considered in patients with SCI who prove appropriate for this technique, especially those who require back-up "demand" pacing rather than continuous pacing.

Tachyarrhythmias

Incidence and etiology: On theoretic grounds, it would be unlikely that the incidence of tachyarrhythmias should be substantially different from that seen in the general population. We have helped confirm this theory by undertaking 24-hour Holter monitoring in 50 patients with SCI. This study showed no higher incidence of tachyarrhythmias in either the high-level or low-level injury group compared to a control population. If tachyarrhythmias are encountered, it is important to document the etiology and underlying cardiovascular status, as these are the two most important determinants of the natural history of this disorder as well as the necessity for initiating treatment.

Atrial fibrillation: This common arrhythmia frequently results from coronary artery disease, long-standing hypertension, and valvular heart disease. Acute treatment depends largely on the rate and hemodynamic response of the patient. If the individual demonstrates significant hemodynamic compromise, then direct current cardioversion should be initiated immediately; this modality is not used frequently enough when warranted. If the patient is stable, then rate control with digoxin, verapamil, or diltiazem is often initiated, with the goal of lowering the heart rate below 100 beats per minute. Beta blockers are also effective for this indication, although they should be used with caution as described above; esmolol may represent a good choice because of its very short half-life. Pharmacologic conversion and prophylaxis may then be considered with antiarrhythmic agents such as amiodarone. In general, it is prudent to anticoagulate a patient with warfarin for at least 2 to 3 weeks before and 2 to 3 weeks after cardioversion unless a strong contraindication exists. Emergent and urgent cardioversion can be done without any form of anticoagulation, although transesophageal echocardiography can be used to rapidly exclude the presence of left atrial mural thrombus, thereby reassuring the practitioner that acute cardioversion is indeed safe. Based upon the results of recent randomized trials, it is desirable to administer chronic warfarin anticoagulation for the majority of patients with chronic atrial fibrillation. Aspirin may represent a viable alternative in individuals with a low risk of embolic stroke or with contraindications to warfarin.

Supraventricular tachyarrhythmias: Patients who present with hemodynamic compromise and/or significant symptoms during a bout of supraventricular tachyarrhythmia (SVT) should be immediately treated with synchronized cardioversion or with bolus adenosine. If the patient is stable, pharmacologic cardioversion is preferable, particularly if non-pharmacologic maneuvers, such as carotid sinus massage, are unsuccessful. Intravenous adenosine is the preferred agent for this group of individuals because of its very short half-life.

Ventricular tachycardia: As with other tachyarrhythmias, the urgency of treatment of ventricular tachycardia lies largely with its effect on overall circulation. Electrical cardioversion should be applied immediately to patients with hemodynamic compromise. If the patient is stable, intravenous lidocaine administered by bolus and continuous infusion should be tried first. Intravenous amiodarone, bretylium and procainamide represent alternative agents. If possible, prior to converting the rhythm, careful documentation of the nature of the rhythm is extremely important and may influence the future evaluation process. Hence, a full 12-lead ECG and rhythm strip is useful, and may be supplemented by carotid sinus massage and/or use of an esophageal lead to help document the origin of the observed wide complex tachycardia (ventricular vs. supraventricular). Also, be sure that electrolyte concentrations (including magnesium) are in the normal range.

Hypotension/Hypertension

Symptomatic hypotension: Profound hypotension is quite common after acute cervical SCI. Although the hypotension generally improves over the ensuing weeks (analogous to the transition from flaccid to spastic paralysis in the somatic nervous system), relatively low blood pressure may continue lifelong. It is important to note that systolic pressures encountered in these young, otherwise healthy individuals with high-level SCI are often impressively low (sometimes in the range of 60 mm Hg–70 mm Hg). This hypotension is particularly noted during changes in position or with standing (as observed during tilt table exercises). Most often, these individuals are asymptomatic despite these low pressures. The improvement in the symptoms of hypotension partially can be attributed to a greater tolerance of low cerebral perfusion pressure, possibly due to resetting of the threshold for cerebral autoregulation. [15] If the hypotension is accompanied by symptoms, several approaches can be applied to help correct this problem. Due to loss of the "buffering" effect of sympathetic tone to the peripheral vasculature, these patients often are quite responsive to changes in position. Therefore, a quick, simple and safe technique to restore arterial pressure is to place the patient in a supine or Trendelenburg position. If unhelpful, a careful fluid challenge should be administered to help exclude the possibility of hypovolemia and underfilling of the ventricles during diastole. This can best be done by carefully checking arterial pressure and pulse, administering up to 500 ml of intravenous fluid as rapidly as possible, and carefully rechecking arterial pressure and pulse rate again. Larger amounts of fluid should be administered only with great caution, if at all. Meyer et al performed hemodynamic studies and blood volume determinations in 9 acutely injured patients with quadriplegia in Vietnam.[16] They found that the observed hypotension is accompanied by a decrease in systemic vascular resistance and actual increase in cardiac output, implicating pathologic vasodilation as the primary disturbance. Unlike their control patients with hemorrhagic shock, clinical resuscitation efforts often led to significant overhydration and overtransfusion. This factor may be responsible for the increased incidence of pulmonary edema noted during spinal shock in this study and others. If hypovolemia is excluded as a cause, then pharmacologic intervention is warranted. Due to the inappropriate vasodilation and high cardiac output state of most patients with high-level SCI with normal cardiac function, the use of inotropic agents is ill advised. As an alternative, selective α- agonists, such as phenylephrine, can be given. Please remember that patients with quadriplegia exhibit a hyperresponsiveness to sympathomimetic agents such as this, and that a low dose should be used at first with a slow titration to the desired effect. Agents such as dopamine might be best reserved for individuals with documented or suspected myocardial dysfunction.

Severe hypertension: Due to the primary disturbance in cardiovascular homeostasis induced by high-level SCI, episodic hypertension as well as hypotension can represent a significant problem. Of particular importance is the syndrome of autonomic dysreflexia, discussed in a separate chapter in this book. We have observed rapid and asymptomatic increases in systolic pressure from 60 mm Hg to 300 mm Hg in some patients with chronic quadriplegia. These extreme changes are generally well tolerated and should not be overtreated, but in aging individuals with cardiovascular disease they may also contribute to significant morbidity and mortality. Therapy should be directed at the rapid and reversible correction of hypertension. You should avoid agents with slow onset and with a persistent effect, to avoid the phenomenon of rebound hypotension after the dysreflexive episode spontaneously abates. Agents such as sublingual nitroglycerin, oral clonidine, parenteral nitroprusside, parenteral hydralazine, and parenteral labetalol have all been used with varying degrees of success. Sublingual nifedipine, used often in the past, should be avoided based on more recent work pointing to frequent adverse outcomes with this drug. Unfortunately, no study to date has documented the ideal treatment for this situation. Please remember that changes in position (such as vertical tilt) often can be helpful and are obviously easily reversible. Also remember that close monitoring is important during a particularly severe episode, as changes in blood pressure may be both quite rapid and quite profound.

References

1. Cushing H. The medical department of the United States Army in the World War. 1927;11:757.

2. Eisenberg M, Tierney D. The aging SCI veteran: a new health care imperative. *VA Practitioner: the magazine for the physicians and pharmacists of the Veterans Administration.* 1985;42-49.

3. Foundation for Spinal Cord Injury. List of Funded Projects 1982-1984. Washington, DC: Paralyzed Veterans of America, Spinal Cord Research Foundation, 1984.

4. Mesard L, Carmody A, Mannarino E, Ruge D. Survival after spinal cord trauma: a life table analysis. *Arch Neurol* 1978;35:78.

5. Sheldon J, Chief Psychosocial Rehabilitation, SCIS, VACO, 6 August 1984, personal communication.

6. Lehmann KG, Lane JG, Piepmeier JM, Batsford WP. Cardiovascular abnormalities accompanying acute spinal cord injury in man: incidence, time course and severity. *J Am Coll Cardiol* 1987;10:46-52.

7. Lehmann KG, Lane JG, Batsford WP. Cardiac rhythm disturbances associated with acute spinal cord injury (abstract). *Circulation* 1984;70:11-15.

8. Piepmeier JM, Lehmann KG, Lane JG. Cardiovascular instability following acute spinal cord trauma. *Cent Nerv Sys Trauma* 1985;2:153.

9. Mathias CJ, Frankel HL, Christensen NJ, Spalding JMK. Enhanced pressor response to noradrenaline in patients with cervical spinal cord transection. *Brain* 1976;99:1757.

10. Christensen NJ, Frankel HL, Mathias CJ, Spalding JMK. Enhanced pressor response to noradrenaline in human subjects with chronic sympathetic decentralization. *J Physiol* 1975;252:39P.

11. Kurnick NB. Autonomic hyperreflexia and its control in patients with spinal cord lesions. *Ann Intern Med* 1956;44:678.

12. Lindan R, Joiner E, Freehafer AA, Hazel C. Incidence and clinical features of autonomic dysreflexia in patients with spinal cord injury. *Paraplegia* 1980;18:285.

13. Shea JD, Gioffre R, Carrion H, Small MP. Autonomic hyperreflexia in spinal cord injury. *South Med J* 1973;66:869.

14. Lehmann KG, Shandling AH, Yusi AU, Froelicher VF. Altered ventricular repolarization in central sympathetic dysfunction from spinal cord injury. *Am J Cardiol* 1989;63:1498-504.

15. Eidelman BH. Cerebral blood flow in normal and abnormal man (Thesis). Oxford, England: University of Oxford 1973.

16. Meyer GA, Berman IR, Doty DB, et al. Hemodynamic responses to acute quadriplegia with or without chest trauma. *J Neurosurg* 1971;34:168.

|PULMONARY COMPLICATIONS

in Chronic SCI

T. Scott Gallacher, MD, MS; C. Kees Mahutte, MD, PhD

CHAPTER THREE ▰▰▰

|Advances in treatment have increased life expectancy in spinal cord injury (SCI) to over 30 years. This has mainly been the result of improved recognition and intervention during the acute injury phase, but has assured a steadily increasing population of individuals in the chronic SCI phase. Despite such advances, common chronic complications include urinary tract infections and decubiti.[1,2] However, the major causes of death in both acute and chronic SCIs are due to pulmonary complications.[3-5] Specifically these include acute respiratory failure, thromboembolism, pneumonia, chronic obstructive pulmonary disease (COPD), bronchitis, sepsis with acute respiratory distress syndrome (ARDS), and lung cancer. Atelectasis and pneumonia are common sequelae of SCI.

|Pulmonary complications are increased in patients with SCI with higher level lesions, reduced spirometry (FEV1 and FVC), impaired gas exchange (lower PaO_2), and advancing age.[1]

Anatomy and Pathophysiology

|The anatomic level of SCI determines the potential extent of pulmonary complications and respiratory muscle compromise. Ventilation is due mainly to diaphragmatic function—innervated primarily by C3, 4, 5—and partially by sternocleidomastoid, scalene, trapezius, and external intercostal muscles. Cough is primarily due to intact function of the abdominal muscles—T6-T12—and internal intercostals (Figure I).

|Upper cervical lesions, C1-C3, result in virtual total respiratory paralysis. Patients are unable to talk, cough, or breathe and require mechanical ventilation. It is sometimes possible for small tidal volumes (60 cc to 300 cc) to be generated by the neck muscles. These may eventually hypertrophy allowing elevation of the sternum and expansion of the upper rib cage, creating tidal volumes over 300 cc. Glossopharyngeal breathing in which small amounts of air can be injected into the trachea using the upper airway muscles including the tongue, cheek, pharyngeal, and laryngeal muscles can be learned. Bilateral phrenic nerve pacemakers have been used to wean these patients from the ventilator, but because of diaphragm atrophy, this intervention must be introduced slowly. Key sequelae of lesions at this level are tracheal intubation requirements, mechanical ventilator dependence, atelectasis, and pneumonia.[6, 7]

|Cervical lesions, C3-C8, usually result in partial to completely normal diaphragmatic function. This function is quite dependent upon patient position—respiration is easier and vital capacity larger in the supine position as the abdominal contents push the diaphragm upwards, placing it at a more mechanically advantageous point from which to begin inspiratory descent. In the sitting position, abdominal binders should be used to improve lung function.[8] Expiratory pressure can be generated by the pectoralis muscles, but often can only affect 50% of normal maximal expiratory flow, which is insufficient for adequate mucus clearance (requires flows of > 5-6 liters/second).[9] The pulmonary function tests of patients with cervical cord lesions typically show a restrictive spirometry pattern with preserved FEV1:FVC ratio and decreased lung volumes (vital capacity, total lung capacity, and expiratory reserve volume) to around 20% to 50% of normal. However, the lung volumes, pressures, inspiratory and expiratory flows correlate poorly with the sensory-motor level of injury and can be quite variable. It is not unusual for improvement in lung function to be seen up to a year after the original injury. The addition of muscle-strengthening programs and, most recently, preliminary studies with anabolic steroids have been shown to result in significant improvements in respiratory function.[10-12] Ventilator-dependent patients with high cervical cord lesions may become weanable.[13]

|Key sequelae of lesions at this level are restrictive lung function, reduced lung and chest wall compliance, inefficient paradoxical breathing (i.e., no chest wall expansion during inspiration due to non-functioning intercostal muscles), and occasional mechanical ventilator requirements.[14,15] The reduced expiratory pressures result in inadequate cough and subsequent retention of secretions and may lead to pneumonia.

|Thoracic cord lesions generally result in less severe changes in lung volumes and inspiratory respiratory muscle strength. However, as these spinal levels are responsible for the major component of expiratory muscle function and cough, key sequelae are retained secretions, mucus plugging, and pneumonia.

|Other anticipated respiratory changes with SCI include bronchoconstriction and increased mucus secretion (due to parasympathetic imbalance from absent sympathetic outflow), increased respiratory rates (typically 14 to 18 breaths per minute in tetraplegia), and recurrent aspiration (contributed to by ileus, vocal cord paralysis, and gastroesophageal reflux). However, in the stable patient, blood gases may be remarkably normal.

Specific Respiratory Complications and Interventions

Secretions: Maintenance of bronchial hygiene is a major problem in patients with SCI and is key to the prevention of further respiratory complications. Expiratory muscle weakness results in decreased ability to cough and consequent retention of secretions. Atelectasis, pneumonia, and respiratory failure will result if aggressive measures are not undertaken to prevent the retention of secretions. The quantity and viscosity of secretions may be increased due to lack of sympathetic nervous system outflow.

|If excessive secretions are present, frequent changes in patient position have been advocated. Recently, this has taken the form of the kinetic treatment table.[5] The traditional wedge-turning device may be going out of vogue, but regardless of how it is done, patient position should be changed frequently (every 2 hours). This should be followed by incentive spirometry at routine intervals (every 4 hours or so), deep breathing exercises, chest percussion, and assisted (quad) cough. If these measures fail to adequately promote the clearance of mucus, then tracheal suctioning, intermittent nebulized or inhaled bronchodilators, or an externally applied pneumatic percussion (ABI) vest can be tried. As the increased viscosity of purulent secretions is due in large part to DNA from lysed inflammatory cells, nebulization of human recombinant Dnase (Pulmozyme) into the airways has been shown effective in clearing purulent secretions.[16]

|Recent research has indicated that stimulation of spinal nerves by application of an external magnetic induction coil is possible and can augment expiratory muscle force.[17,18] A device of this sort may prove useful in the future for promoting cough and expectoration of secretions in patients with SCI.

Atelectasis: If the previously mentioned measures to remove secretions and prevent atelectasis have been unsuccessful, a variety of approaches may be tried to re-expand atelectatic lung areas. It should be remembered that persistent atelectasis can occur despite all measures and if gas exchange remains acceptable, the patient may have to live with a permanently collapsed lobe.

|Suggested approaches to atelectasis would include simply waiting, percussion, or directed suctioning. Directional tip-curved suction catheters are available to suction the left lung airways (because the left mainstem bronchus branches at an acute angle from the trachea). Flexible fiberoptic bronchoscopy may be required to remove secretions from lung segments out of reach of the suction catheter. Direct visualization of the airways is important in refractory atelectasis because patients with SCI may still have risk factors for endobronchial lesions and lung cancer. Bronchoscopy also allows direct instillation of mucolytic agents into the atelectatic area and may facilitate lung re-expansion. All such suctioning measures are not without problem. Mechanical damage to mucociliary clearance mechanisms can occur and leads to a vicious cycle of recurrent secretions and atelectasis. Repeated bronchoscopy may become self-defeating and would not be indicated.

|In the tracheally intubated patient, the judicious use of positive end-expiratory pressure (PEEP) provides the best means of opening the atelectatic lobe. Because PEEP effects depend on the degree of lung compliance, differential effects, such as overdistention of the non-atelectatic lung, can occur. Double-lumen endotracheal intubation and differential lung ventilation have been tried, but are generally not recommended due to difficulty in maintaining these special endotracheal tubes. These tubes tend to become malpositioned frequently. In addition, their small lumen hampers adequate removal of secretions.

Airway resistance: Not only can bronchoconstriction be caused by parasympathetic nervous system imbalance, but airway resistance can be increased by secretions or underlying conditions such as COPD or asthma. Bronchodilators may be given via nebulizer or metered dose inhaler if increases in airway resistance are recognized.Such medications can also improve mucociliary clearance. Typical bronchodilators are beta-2 sympathetic agonists, but ipratropium bromide (useful in COPD) can also be used with the added effect of a slight decrease in pulmonary secretions. Theophylline is a useful bronchodilator and also improves mucociliary clearance. There is some evidence that theophylline and aminopyridine compounds may also improve diaphragmatic contractility and reduce fatigue, but these pharmacological effects are probably clinically insignificant.[19] A single study of oxybutynin suggests a possible mechanism (cholinergic pathways) of airway hyperreactivity in patients with SCI.[20]

Respiratory muscle function: Respiratory muscles that may be weakened by the primary neurologic injury itself can be easily fatigued by the increased resistive or elastic loads imposed by secretions, bronchospasm, atelectasis, pneumonia, or effusions often seen in patients with SCI. It has been demonstrated that inspiratory resistive training for 30 minutes each day can improve respiratory muscle strength and endurance and may even be useful in weaning patients from ventilators. Appropriate training programs can also strengthen the clavicular head of the pectoralis major muscle that improves expiratory muscle performance.[10,11] Improved bronchial hygiene and an improved ability to deal with loads on the respiratory system can result from such training of inspiratory and expiratory muscles.

|Useful adjuncts may also be pharmacological. Evidence exists that theophylline improves diaphragmatic contractility. More recently anabolic steroids (oxandrolone, 20 mg/day for 1 month in patients with tetraplegia) have been found to reduce the incidence of pulmonary complications by causing general weight gain, decreased ratings of dyspnea (Borg score), and improving spirometry (maximal inspiratory and expiratory pressures).[12]

Pneumonia: Inadequate cough and retention of secretions frequently leads to pneumonia in patients with SCI. The incidence of pneumonia can vary from 6% to 38% in acute SCI to between 1% to 6% at annual follow-up evaluations. [21,22] Initial presentation may show an increased respiratory rate as the lone objective finding. Additional clinical manifestations, such as fever, dyspnea, purulent sputum, and diminished breath sounds, also occur. The physical examination may be difficult due to the patient's inability to inspire deeply.

|Aspiration also occurs. Empiric antibiotic coverage should therefore be aggressive and cover both Gram-positive and Gram-negative organisms including anaerobes. Ineffectively treated pneumonia can progress to acute respiratory distress syndrome (ARDS) and septic shock. The typical hemodynamic profile of septic shock (high cardiac output and low peripheral vascular resistance) may be seen in the stable, non-septic patient with SCI and may lead to some confusion. Besides appropriate antibiotics, the usual treatments with fluids and vasopressors should be undertaken.

Acute respiratory failure: All of the aforementioned complications can lead to acute respiratory failure as can other problems (such as pneumothorax and pulmonary embolism) that impair gas exchange. Acute respiratory failure is characterized by a decreased PaO_2 (gas exchange) and /or an increased $PaCO_2$ (impaired ventilation and muscle fatigue). Because patients with SCI have so many potential pulmonary problems, the significance of these changes may go unrecognized resulting in acute mechanical ventilatory requirements, decompensation, and death.

|It can be surmised from the intensity of respiratory care that patients with SCI require, that a close partnership between all caregivers (physicians, respiratory therapists, nurses, physiotherapists, laboratory and radiology staff, etc.) is essential. If individual pulmonary complications are inadequately prevented or treated, a cascade of respiratory compromise will ensue resulting in acute respiratory failure (Figure II). Mechanisms to promptly assess the severity of gas exchange impairment must be in place and appropriate interventions readily available. Acute respiratory failure is a terminal event for many patients with SCI.

ARDS: ARDS is characterized by leaky pulmonary capillaries, pulmonary edema, severe hypoxemia, bilateral infiltrates on chest X-ray, and decreased lung compliance. In patients with SCI, this may occur in a variety of catastrophic settings including sepsis (often due to decubiti or urinary tract infection), pneumonia, or aspiration. ARDS has also been recognized during the acute stage of SCI perhaps due to increased catecholamine release seen in the context of severe neurologic insult.[23,24]

|Treatment consists of eliminating the precipitating cause and ventilatory support. A consensus has developed, indicating that patients with ARDS should be ventilated with low tidal volumes (6 to 8 ml/kg), optimal PEEP, and limited static inflation pressures (less than 35 cm H_2O). Gas exchange may also be improved by placing the patient in the prone position. There is no convincing evidence that improving oxygen transport influences mortality. The overall mortality in ARDS remains at 40% to 60%. Steroids and most other "innovative" therapies (immunomodulators, selective pulmonary vasodilators, surfactant, etc.) have not proven useful in reducing acute ARDS mortality. However, if ARDS persists (so-called late-stage or fibro-proliferative-phase ARDS), systemic corticosteroids may have some utility.

Pleural effusions: In the patients with SCI, pleural effusions are most often parapneumonic. They complicate around 40% of bacterial pneumonias and are exudative—pleural fluid:serum protein ratio 0.5, or pleural fluid LDH:serum LDH ratio >0.6, or pleural fluid LDH > ⅔ upper limit of normal for serum. They may also result from renal failure, pulmonary embolus, or intra-abdominal processes. In the setting of acute SCI, chylothorax and hemothorax should also be considered. Eosinophilic effusions can result from a variety of medications—typical examples are nitrofurantoin, used in the treatment of urinary tract infections, and dantrolene, used to treat spasticity. Pleuropulmonary reactions can also occur with methysergide, bromocriptine, procarbazine, and amiodarone.

|Treatment of pleural effusions is similar to those occurring in able-bodied individuals and indications for chest-tube drainage and pleurodesis are no different. The major difficulties in dealing with pleural effusions in patients with SCI involve the performance of the diagnostic tests themselves. Frequently routine chest X-ray evaluations (AP, semi-recumbent views) are barely adequate to visualize even significant pleural effusions, and special views (decubitus) may be physically impossible. Likewise, in attempting thoracentesis, positioning the patient appropriately may not be possible and concurrent medical therapies, such as chronic anticoagulation, may hamper the prompt performance of such invasive interventions. It is crucial to consider pleural effusion in the differential diagnosis of difficult ventilator weaning and gas exchange abnormalities. The work-up may require computer-aided tomography (CT) scan delineation of the pleural effusion and ultrasound guidance in thoracentesis attempts.

Sleep apnea: Sleep apnea is uncommon in young patients with SCI. There is a suggestion that the incidence increases with age in males, but data are scarce.[25,26] Monitoring with pulse oximetry may detect nocturnal arterial oxygen desaturations, and clinical evidence of sleep apnea (snoring, daytime somnolence, morning headaches, etc.) should be sought.

|A special situation exists in patients with tetraplegia with an elevated $PaCO_2$ and decreased ventilatory response to CO_2. In these patients, alveolar hypoventilation may worsen with sleep resulting in increases in $PaCO_2$ and accompanied by oxygen desaturation.

|Suspicion of sleep apnea should prompt performance of polysomnography in an accredited sleep laboratory. Due to the logistics of bringing some patients with SCI into the sleep laboratory, portable monitoring of pulse oximetry, snoring, and airflows can be used to document nocturnal airflow obstruction and oxygen desaturation. It can also be used to assess response to treatment. This method is somewhat unsatisfactory because no information about sleep EEG or muscle tone is obtained.

|Treatment of sleep apnea or nocturnal oxygen desaturation consists of traditional measures (nasal continuous positive airway pressure, nasal bi-level positive airway pressure, supplemental oxygen, tracheotomy, etc.).

Pulmonary embolism: Deep venous thrombosis (DVT) is a common occurrence and can lead to fatal pulmonary embolism.[27-29] The greatest risk is within the first 3 to 6 months of acute SCI and may include associations unique to the patient with SCI (e.g., DVT from ankle orthoses).[30] Conventional prevention and treatment of DVT is indicated at least during the first 3 to 6 months after SCI. Current DVT prophylaxis recommendations seem to be applicable to patients with SCI although specific studies in patients with SCI are limited. The use of low molecular weight heparins (e.g., Enoxaparin) has been advocated.[31,32] During the chronic phase of SCI the incidence of DVT and pulmonary embolism is seen to decrease and the routine continuation of anticoagulation may not be necessary.[33]

|In patients with chronic SCI with a prior history of DVT and new limb swelling, the diagnosis of new DVT may be difficult. Traditional venous Doppler ultrasound examinations may be positive and unable to distinguish between old vs. new DVT. This is particularly problematic because patients with SCI tend to recanalize lower extremity veins more slowly than ambulatory individuals. Full anticoagulation for "recurrent DVT" may be indicated even without a definite diagnosis.

|Perhaps the most significant problem in the diagnosis of pulmonary embolism in these patients is that it is frequently misdiagnosed as pneumonitis or atelectasis. A ventilation perfusion scan may not reliably differentiate between these conditions, and adjunctive measures (such as D-dimer evaluation) may be required.[34, 35] A spiral contrast enhanced CT scan may be ordered as it can often show large pulmonary emboli. Occasionally patients with SCI may proceed to bronchoscopy to eliminate the possibility of atelectasis due to mucus plugging. False-positive, perfusion-only lung scans have been described in a few patients with SCI with normal pulmonary angiograms—these particular patients responded to improved pulmonary toilet.

|In patients with SCI who fail anticoagulation, vena-caval interruption ("Greenfield filter") is indicated. If this device is placed, thereafter assisted ("quad") coughing is contraindicated because displacement and migration of the vena-caval filter can occur.[36]

Late-onset ventilatory failure: Although many individuals with high cervical cord injuries are successfully weaned from mechanical ventilation, a few may experience late-onset ventilatory failure. This should be suspected in patients with unexplained tachypnea, dyspnea, daytime somnolence, erythrocytosis, sleep apnea, fluctuating mental alertness, and respiratory muscle fatigue with increased positional influences on breathing.

|Late-onset ventilatory failure may be due to late neurologic decline as seen in compression with cervical stenosis and post-traumatic syringomyelia. It can be complicated by obesity, recurrent atelectasis or pneumonia, progressive scoliosis or kyphosis, and aging (loss of diaphragmatic motor neurons).

|Evaluation is necessary to assess for potentially treatable etiologies and to confirm the extent of respiratory failure. Interventions would obviously include supporting ventilation (CPAP, BiPAP, oxygen supplementation, tracheotomy, mechanical ventilation) and preventing further decline in respiratory function by discontinuing cigarette smoking and instituting a program of respiratory muscle strengthening and bronchial hygiene. Teaching glossopharyngeal breathing may be of some use in maintaining tidal volumes.

Conclusion

|SCI is a significant problem worldwide. It impacts on individual quality of life, and has a financial impact on health care.[37-42] Overall mortality is improving and current spinal cord research shows promise.[43]

|However, the major cause of morbidity and mortality continues to be pulmonary problems. These complications can be predicted on the basis of the spinal level of injury and the approach to these pulmonary concerns can be algorithmic.

Go PhAAR for CPR in SCI.

Go PhAAR (far): attend to phlegm, avoid atelectasis, and treat airway resistance.

C — cord level to predict pulmonary needs (e.g., ventilator or not)

P — prevention of pneumonia and respiratory failure/ARDS. To accomplish this, you must have

R — respiratory muscle training

The pulmonary concerns of these patients would also include SCI.

S — sleep. Unrecognized sleep apnea or nocturnal hypoventilation is problematic.

C — clotting. Acute DVT and pulmonary embolism follow traditional recommendations, but patients with chronic SCI demand different approaches.

I — impaired gas exchange and iatrogenesis. Usual clinical evaluations may underestimate significance of gas exchange abnormalities and various medications can result in pleural effusions, hypoventilation, etc.

Figure I **Guide to Cord Level Damage**

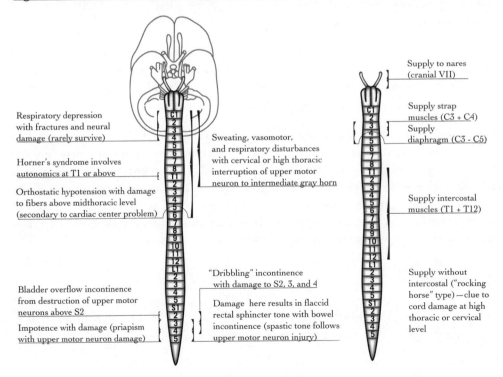

Respiratory depression with fractures and neural damage (rarely survive)

Horner's syndrome involves autonomics at T1 or above

Orthostatic hypotension with damage to fibers above midthoracic level (secondary to cardiac center problem)

Bladder overflow incontinence from destruction of upper motor neurons above S2

Impotence with damage (priapism with upper motor neuron damage)

Sweating, vasomotor, and respiratory disturbances with cervical or high thoracic interruption of upper motor neuron to intermediate gray horn

"Dribbling" incontinence with damage to S2, 3, and 4

Damage here results in flaccid rectal sphincter tone with bowel incontinence (spastic tone follows upper motor neuron injury)

Supply to nares (cranial VII)

Supply strap muscles (C3 + C4)

Supply diaphragm (C3 - C5)

Supply intercostal muscles (T1 + T12)

Supply without intercostal ("rocking horse" type) — clue to cord damage at high thoracic or cervical level

EMERGENCIES

*Edited by: Ibrahim M. Eltorai, MD
and James K. Schmitt, MD
Foreword by: Joel A. DeLisa, MD, MS*

in Chronic Spinal Cord Injury Patients

3RD EDITION

The editors would like to draw your attention to
the following corrections.

Page 69, line 33, first word should read Sudomotor.

Page 138, line 16, fourth word should read homocystinemia.

Figure II **Development of ARF**

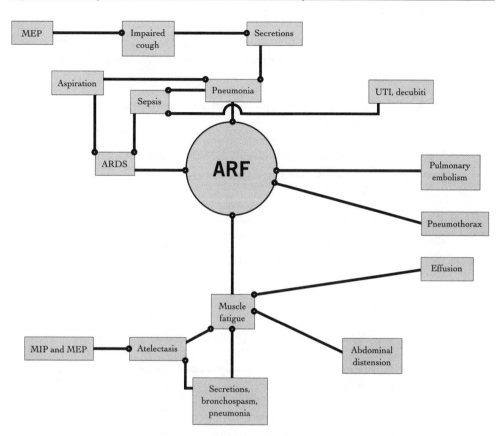

References

1. Reines HD, Harris RC. Pulmonary complications of acute spinal cord injuries. *Neurosurgery* 1987;21(2):193-196.

2. Spungen AM, Grimm DR, Lesser M, et al. Self-reported prevalence of pulmonary symptoms in subjects with spinal cord injury. *Spinal Cord* 1997;35:652-657.

3. Lucke KT. Pulmonary management following acute SCI. *J Neuroscience Nursing* 1998;30(2):91-104.

4. Viroslav J, Rosenblatt R, Tomazevic SM. Respiratory management, survival, and quality of life for high-level traumatic tetraplegics. *Respir Care Clin N Am* 1996;2(2):313-322.

5. Borkowski C. A comparison of pulmonary complications in spinal cord-injured patients treated with two modes of spinal immobilization. *J Neurosci Nurs* 1989;21(2):79-85.

6. Fromm B, Hunt G, Gemer HJ, et al. Management of respiratory problems unique to high tetraplegia. *Spinal Cord* 1999;37(4):239-244.

7. Fujiwara T, Hara Y, Chino N. Expiratory function in complete tetraplegics: study of spirometry, maximal expiratory pressure, and muscle activity of pectoralis major and latissimus dorsi muscles. *Am J Phys Med Rehabil* 1999;78(5):464-469.

8. Estenne M, Van Muylem A, Gorini M, et al. Effects of abdominal strapping on forced expiration in tetraplegic patients. *Am J Respir Crit Care Med* 1998;157(1):95-98.

9. Gounden P. Static respiratory pressures inpatients with post-traumatic tetraplegia. *Spinal Cord* 1997;35(1):43-47.

10. Uijl SG, Houtman S, Folgering HT, Hopman MT. Training of the respiratory muscles in individuals with tetraplegia. *Spinal Cord* 1999;37(8):575-579.

11. Rutchik A, Weissman AR, Almenoff PL, et al. Resistive inspiratory muscle training in subjects with chronic cervical spinal cord injury. *Arch Phys Med Rehabil* 1998;79(3):293-297.

12. Spungen AM, Grimm DR, Strakhan M, et al. Treatment with an anabolic agent is associated with improvement in respiratory function in persons with tetraplegia: a pilot study. *Mt Sinai J Med* 1999;66(3):201-205.

13. Peterson WP, Barbalata L, Brooks CA, Gerhart KA, et al. The effect of tidal volumes on the time to wean persons with high tetraplegia from ventilators. *Spinal Cord* 1999;37(4):284-288.

14. Lin KH, Chuang CC, Wu HD, et al. Abdominal weight and inspiratory resistance: their immediate effects on inspiratory muscle functions during maximal voluntary breathing in chronic tetraplegic patients. *Arch Phys Med Rehabil* 1999;80(7):741-745.

15. Blackmer J, Marshall S. Obesity and spinal cord injury: an observational study. *Spinal Cord* 1997;35(4):245-247.

16. Voelker KG, Chetty KG, Mahutte CK. Resolution of recurrent atelectasis in spinal cord injury patients with administration of recombinant human DNase. *Intensive Care Medicine* 1996;22:582-584.

17. Lin VWH, Singh H, Chitkara RK, Perkash I. Functional magnetic stimulation for restoring cough in patients with tetraplegia. *Arch Phys Med Rehabil* 1998;79:517-522.

18. Polkey MI, Luo Y, Guliera R, Hamnegard CH, et al. Functional magnetic stimulation of the abdominal muscles in humans. *Am J Respir Crit Care Med* 1999;160(2):513-522.

19. Segal JL, Brunnemann SR. 4-Aminopyridine improves pulmonary function in quadriplegic humans with longstanding spinal cord injury. *Pharmacotherapy* 1997;17(3):415-423.

20. Singas E, Grimm DR, Almenoff PL, Lesser M. Inhibition of airway hyperreactivity by oxybutynin chloride in subjects with cervical spinal cord injury. *Spinal Cord* 1999;37(4):279-283.

21. Berrouane Y, Daudenthun I, Riegel B, et al. Early onset pneumonia in neurosurgical intensive care unit patients. *J Hosp Infect* 1998;40(4):275-280.

22. Montgomerie JZ. Infections in patients with spinal cord injuries. *Clin Infect Dis* 1997;25(6):1285-1290.

23. Atkinson JLD. The neglected prehospital phase of head injury: apnea and the catecholamine surge. *Mayo Clinic Proc* 2000;75:37-47.

24. Chiou-Tan FY, Eisele SG, Song JX. Increased norepinephrine levels during catheterization inpatients with spinal cord injury. *Am J Phys Med Rehabil* 1999;78(4):350-353.

25. Klefbeck B, Sternhag M, Weinberg J, et al. Obstructive sleep apneas in relation to severity of cervical spinal cord injury. *Spinal Cord* 1998;36(9):621-628.

26. Mello MT, Silva AC, Rueda AD, et al. Correlation between K complex, periodic leg movements (PLM), and myoclonus during sleep in paraplegic adults before and after an acute physical activity. *Spinal Cord* 1997;35(4):248-252.

27. Green D, Hull RD, Mammen EF, Merli GJ, et al. Deep vein thrombosis in spinal cord injury: summary and recommendations. *Chest* 1992;102 (6 suppl): 633S-635S.

28. Britt LD, Zolfaghari D, Kennedy E, et al. Incidence and prophylaxis of deep vein thrombosis in a high risk trauma population. *Am J Surg* 1996;172(1):13-14.

29. Gallus AS, Nurmohammed M, Kearon C, Prins M. Thromboprophylaxis in non-surgical patients: who, when and how? *Haemostasis* 1998;28(Suppl)3:71-82.

30. Kroll HR, Odderson IR, Allen FH. Deep vein thrombi associated with the use of plastic ankle-foot orthoses. *Arch Phys Med Rehabil* 1998;79(5):576-578.

31. Tomaio A, Kirshblum SC, O'Connor KC. Treatment of acute deep vein thrombosis in spinal cord injured patients with enoxaparin: a cost analysis. *Spinal Cord Med* 1998;21(3):205-210.

32. Harris S, Chen D, Green D. Enoxaparin for thromboembolism prophylaxis in spinal injury: preliminary report on experience with 105 patients. *Am J Phys Med Rehabil* 1996;75(5):326-327.

33. Scott MP, Jezic GA, Swenson JR. Calf vein thrombosis in spinal cord injured patients: conservative management of two cases. *Arch Phys Med Rehabil* 1997;78(5):538-539.

34. More O'Ferrall DJ, Cohn JR, Rider-Foster D. False positive perfusion lung scintiscans in tetraplegic patients: a case series. *Arch Phys Med Rehabil* 1999;80(10):1343-1345.

35. Roussi J, Bentolila S, Boudaoud L, et al. Contribution of D-Dimer determination in the exclusion of deep venous thrombosis in spinal cord injury patients. *Spinal Cord* 1999;37(8):548-552.

36. Greenfield LJ. Does cervical spinal cord injury induce a higher incidence of complications after prophylactic Greenfield filter usage? [letter; comment] Comment on: *J Vasc Interv Radiol* 1996;7(6):907-915. *J Vasc Interv Radiol* 1997;8(4):719-720.

37. Westgren N, Levi R. Quality of life and traumatic spinal cord injury. *Arch Phys Med Rehabil* 1998;79(11):1433-1439.

38. McKinley WO, Kolakowsky SA, Kreutzer JS. Substance abuse, violence, and outcome after traumatic spinal cord injury. *Am J Phys Med Rehabil* 1999;78(4):306-312.

39. Botel U, Glaser E, Niedeggen A, Meindl R. The cost of ventilator-dependent spinal cord injuries-patients in the hospital and at home. *Spinal Cord* 1997;35(1):40-42.

40. Bach JR, Rajaraman R, Ballanger F, et al. Neuromuscular ventilatory insufficiency: effect of home mechanical ventilator use v oxygen therapy on pneumonia and hospitalization rates. *Am J Phys Med Rehabil* 1998;77(1):8-19.

41. Tromans AM, Mecci M, Barrett FH, et al. The use of the BiPAP biphasic positive airway pressure system in acute spinal cord injury. *Spinal Cord* 1998;36(7):481-484.

42. Lurie S. Chest Physicians explore worldwide use of home mechanical ventilation. *JAMA* 1999;282:2107-2108.

43. Marwick C. Spinal cord injury research shows promise. *JAMA* 1999;282:2108-2110.

The
SCI VENTILATOR-DEPENDENT PATIENT
Troubleshooting

Diane L. Huntington, RRT

CHAPTER FOUR

When a patient with spinal cord injury (SCI) who is ventilator-dependent comes into the hospital one of the first things that needs to be done is a respiratory assessment. Assessment is not unusual for the medical staff, but having the patient come in on a ventilator may be a new situation. Some of the same questions still pertain whether the patient is breathing spontaneously or being mechanically ventilated. The questions include: Is the patient in respiratory distress? What is the respiratory rate? What is the breathing pattern? Can the patient talk to you? If the patient is capable of speech, how is his breathing? Does he feel like he's having trouble breathing? Does the ventilator feel like it always does to the patient? Does he think there is a problem with the ventilator?

|Most patients on long-term mechanical ventilation have a tracheostomy tube. The majority of home ventilator patients use a cuffless tracheostomy tube so they can talk freely. This works out well as long as the patient is not in any type of acute respiratory distress. If the patient is in respiratory distress, it is recommended that the cuffless tracheostomy tube immediately be changed to a cuffed tracheostomy tube. This is to ensure adequate ventilation and also to monitor the patient's respiratory status more accurately. You can tell if the patient has a cuffed tracheostomy tube by looking for a pilot balloon hanging down from the tracheostomy tube itself. If the tracheostomy tube is changed to a cuffed tube, the tidal volume needs to be adjusted on the ventilator. A patient who has a cuffless tracheostomy tube requires a higher set tidal volume on the ventilator to compensate for the leak. The leak of air around the tube enables him to talk. With an inflated cuff on the tracheostomy tube there won't be a leak. This may very well over-ventilate the patient, unless the machine tidal volume is decreased. An arterial blood gas should be obtained as soon as possible if the patient is having respiratory distress.

|The tracheostomy tube needs to be looked at very carefully. Is the tracheostomy tube patent? If not, does it have an inner cannula that can be taken out to see if it is occluded? Can a suction catheter be passed? If there is still a blockage and the patient is in respiratory distress, deflate the tracheostomy tube cuff (if present) and reposition the tube. Afterwards, inflate the cuff and see if you feel or hear air movement. If not, another tracheostomy tube needs to be re-inserted. Again, it is imperative that if the patient is in respiratory distress a cuffed tracheostomy tube, usually of the same size, needs to be inserted, as long as the patient can be sufficiently suctioned. If another tracheostomy tube of the same size cannot be re-inserted, try the next smaller size. Rarely there is still an occlusion after a new tracheostomy tube has been inserted. In this case a small endotracheal tube can be inserted or an extra long tracheostomy tube can be tried to bypass the obstruction.

|After dealing with the tracheostomy tube, various components of the ventilator should be addressed. Questions that should be asked when dealing with a ventilator are: Is the patient in synchrony with the ventilator? Are there any alarms sounding on the ventilator? Is the staff familiar with this type of ventilator? As always, priority needs to be determined, and if the patient is in respiratory distress or failure, you need to ventilate the patient immediately. Take the patient off the mechanical ventilator and manually ventilate him. Never assume the ventilator is working properly until someone can verify this. This is especially true if the patient is not alert and cannot tell you the status of the ventilator. If the patient can talk or communicate, and is not in respiratory distress ask the patient or caregiver what the ventilator settings are. Verify this by checking to see how the control knobs are set. If the patient states that something just feels different with the ventilator, ask him if there have been any recent changes? Is the tubing new? Has the tubing been changed recently? Does he have a new caregiver? Have any of the methods or procedures relating to his tracheostomy tube or ventilator been changed. The patient who uses a home-ventilator usually knows himself and his equipment extremely well and often directs his care and the training of his caregivers. The longer the patient has had his SCI, the better he knows himself. Therefore, he knows when something is not right. Taking the time to really listen to what the patient is saying may save time and trouble in the long run.

GASTROINTESTINAL

R. Kannan Rajan, MD; Bernard A. Nemchausky, MD

Emergencies in Patients With SCI

CHAPTER FIVE ■■■■■■■■■■■■■■■■

Spinal cord injury (SCI) covers many aspects of medicine and surgery that involve each of the various specialties and subspecialties that impinge on the care of SCI. Spinal medicine continues to be an underdeveloped clinical science. Despite the newer advances in neurophysiology, diagnostic radiology (CT scan, spiral CT, virtual colonoscopy, MR), nuclear medicine, ultrasonography, EUS, EGD, colonoscopy, MRCP and beyond, complexities of spinal medicine—particularly of gastroenterology—pose a formidable challenge to the practicing clinician.

|Hippocrates, in his treatise on the sacred disease, epilepsy, wrote "And man ought to know that from nothing else but the brain comes joys, delights, laughter, and sport, and sorrow, grief, despondency, and lamentations. And by this, in an especial manner, we acquire wisdom and knowledge . . . and by the same organ we become mad and delirious and fears and terrors assail us . . ." All these things a person who is paralyzed endures with an intact brain and a disrupted spinal and peripheral nervous system that deprives him of the use of his extremities and leaves him devoid of somatic pain, which is the most common symptom present in any disease. Pain is essential for the preservation of life. It is the dichotomy of the nervous system between an intact brain and neurogenic dysfunction of the body and limbs that adds to the complexities of clinical presentation and physical findings in spinal cord medicine.

|In order to properly understand the gastrointestinal (GI) emergencies in the patient who is paralyzed, one must realize that the GI function is not only under the major influences of the central, peripheral, autonomic, and enteric nervous systems, but is also greatly influenced by emotional and psychological factors.

|GI diseases are diverse in patients with SCI and this section presents basic principles in recognition and management of GI emergencies. Table I presents axioms in spinal cord medicine and Table II classifies acute GI emergencies in patients with SCI.

Nervous System of Gut
|The central nervous system (CNS) and peripheral nervous system (PNS) control GI function. The PNS is made up of the somatic and autonomic nervous system, both contributing richly to the enteric nervous system (ENS) located in the wall of the bowel.[1] Control mechanisms of the alimentary system reside in the CNS and are mediated through efferent nerves (PNS) that connect the brain to the gut (ENS). Smooth muscle organs like the intestines have a dual innervation, one being excitatory and the other inhibitory. In addition, smooth muscles exhibit inherent spontaneous contractions that are tonic, phasic, or both, independent of CNS, PNS, or ENS control. In the digestive tract, the parasympathetic (cholinergic) nerves are excitatory and the sympathetic (adrenergic) nerves are inhibitory. Symptoms of GI disturbances of the neural control are thought to originate from regional changes in contractile activity. Delayed gastric emptying may be the result of dysfunctional colonic contraction. Incontinence is due to anal sphincter dysfunction.

|The extrinsic innervation of the gut consists of the parasympathetic vagal and sacral nerves (S2, 3, 4) through the pelvic nerves and the sympathetic outflow from the spinal cord, between the levels of T5 and L3 segments (Figure I). The sympathetic nerves synapse in the celiac and mesenteric ganglia. The areas of neural supply generally correspond to the vascular arterial supply. Somatic nerves control the striated muscle portion of the esophagus and external anal sphincter. The gut smooth muscle can function without neural control, but extrinsic nerves are known to assist in the intrinsic control and to integrate activity in disparate areas of the gut. Extrinsic nerves are more important in control of stomach and distal colon than the small bowel (fore and hindgut vs. midgut). Uninhibited vagal activity results in sphincter contraction that may not relax in response to stimuli.

|The ENS on its own constitutes the intrinsic nervous system of the gut. It is distinct and differs from other divisions of the PNS, not only in its complexity but also in its autonomy, and has been rightly termed the brain of the GI tract. It consists of the intramural extension of extrinsic nerve terminals and the intramural neurons with their processes. It is connected to the CNS by sympathetic and parasympathetic nerves. The enteric system is formed by five networks of neurons and their processes, two major and three minor. The two major ganglionated plexuses are the myenteric (Auerbach's) plexuses and the submucous (Meissner's) plexuses. The three minor plexuses are the subserous, the deep myenteric, and mucosal. The mucosal plexuses are further characterized as subglandular, intraglandular, or intravillous mucosal plexuses, depending on their location in the mucosa.

|In addition, the neuroendocrine cells and amine precursor uptake and decarboxylation (APUD) cells in the gut secrete hormones, amines and other neuroregulators of the GI system.[2] The role of intraluminal factors—mechanical, chemical, and biological—on the ENS is complex and depends on specificity of receptors for different types of stimuli.

|In order to appreciate the GI emergencies, one should have a sound knowledge of the pathophysiology of the common GI symptoms, i.e., abdominal pain, nausea, vomiting, constipation, diarrhea, flatulence, and belching.

Abdominal Pain
|Abdominal pain or distress is the most common presenting symptom. It is the dominant symptom of acute abdomen. Pain is subjective, and patients differ greatly in their tolerance of it and their ability to precisely characterize it. The description of pain, its intensity, location, precipitating, aggravating and alleviating factors, and its relation to meals, defecation, and body position are all important in evaluating any disease process.

|Pain stimuli activate a specific set of free nerve endings of small A-delta and C-afferent fibers. Despite the clear morphologic delineation of pain pathways, little is understood about abdominal pain production. It may be due either to activation of pain receptors directly or lowering of threshold to painful stimuli. In inflammation, chemical mediators such as histamine, prostaglandins, and kinins, and in peptic ulcer disease smooth muscle contractions and hydrochloric acid (HCl) are believed to cause pain. The distension of hollow viscus may mediate abnormal colic of bowel obstruction. Delayed transit of intestinal gas, rather than an increase in its volume, probably causes the discomfort of flatulence.

Figure I **Diagram of Visceral Innervation**

Thick solid lines are parasympathetic fibers; the dotted lines represent sympathetic fibers. Preganglionic neurons are shown as solid lines; postganglionic neurons as dotted lines.

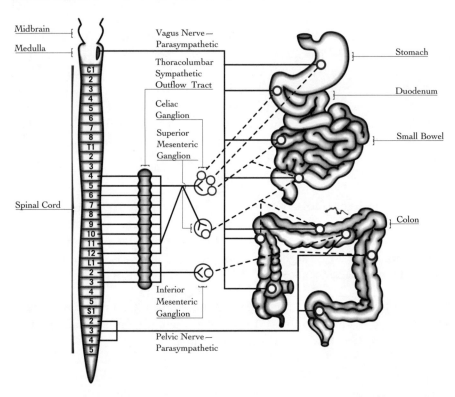

(From: Gore RM, Mintzer RA. *Gastrointestinal Complications: Radiology of Spinal Cord Injury* Calenoff L (Ed). C.V. Mosby Company: St. Louis, 1981.)

|There are three distinct categories of abdominal pain: somatic (parietal), visceral (splanchnic), and referred pain. Basic understanding of these pain responses will help the clinician greatly in evaluating acute abdominal emergencies.

Visceral Pain

|Visceral pain receptors are autonomic nerves in serosal structures of the visceral peritoneum and the capsules of the solid organs, in the mucosa and in the mesentery. Four general classes of stimuli initiate visceral pain: contraction and distension, compression, traction and torsion, stretch and certain chemicals. Visceral pain is felt in mid-line of the abdomen. ENS plays no part in visceral pain perception.

|Description of visceral pain varies from patient to patient with the same disease process. The pain may be characterized as crampy, colicky, gaseous, dull, burning, tearing, squeezing, aching, etc. Visceral pain is perhaps the earliest subtle harbinger of intra-abdominal disease, but because it is ill-defined, diffuse, and poorly localized, it plays minor role in diagnosis in patients with SCI. When it becomes supplanted by somatic pain, it helps greatly in diagnosis.

Somatic Pain

|Parietal nerves in the peritoneum sense pain when irritated by chemical or bacterial influences inside the abdomen. It is sharp, constant, and precisely localized.

Referred Pain

|When the undersurface of the diaphragm is irritated by inflammatory exudate of inflamed abdominal viscus, pain is transmitted by sensory terminations of the phrenic nerve (C3, 4, 5) of the diaphragm to the skin overlying the acromial process innervated by the supraclavicular nerve (Sensory C3, 4). This could occur in acute cholecystitis, although it is unusual. Referred shoulder tip pain is common in gastric or duodenal ulcer perforations. The pain from diaphragmatic irritation, due to subphrenic collection of pus or blood, often radiates to supra clavicular area. Kehr's sign, pain, or possibly hyperesthesia, referred to the left shoulder may occur in ruptured spleen, where effused blood irritates the undersurface of the diaphragm. The pain of ureteral colic often radiates to the lower quadrants, genitalia, or inner thigh. In appendicitis, the initial pain reported is periumbilical or epigastric. Afterwards, it localizes to the right lower quadrant when appendicial inflammation and distension irritates the surrounding parietal peritoneum. This is elicited as McBurney's point tenderness.

Nausea and Vomiting

|Nausea is an unpleasant sensation that may or may not lead to vomiting. Retching and vomiting are separate motor acts involving the somatic muscles (intercostals and diaphragm) and muscle groups involved in posturing as well as smooth muscles in the GI tract and oropharynx. Retching does not always result in vomiting.

|Nausea and vomiting are invariably associated with GI emergencies—peritonitis secondary to perforated viscus, small bowel obstruction or pseudo-obstruction, gastric volvulus, gallstone ileus, etc. Retching and vomiting are less common in people with quadriplegia.

GI emergencies: GI emergencies in patients with SCI are not any different from the ones in the general population except in their clinical presentation. The most common GI emergencies are:

    I. GI bleeding
    II. Acute abdomen
        A. Paralytic ileus (adynamic ileus)
        B. Bowel obstruction
            i. Gastro-duodenal obstruction
            ii. Small bowel obstruction
            iii. Large bowel obstruction
        C. Acute peptic ulcer perforation
            i. Perforation of other viscera
        D. Inflammatory process
            i. Appendicitis
            ii. Cholecystitis
            iii. Pancreatitis
        E. Blunt trauma to abdomen
        F. Peritonitis
        G. Intra-abdominal Abscess
            i. Liver abscess
            ii. Pancreatic abscess
            iii. Subphrenic abscess
            iv. Ischio-rectal abscess
        H. Urologic causes
            i. Pyelonephritis
            ii. Cystitis
            iii. Renal and perirenal abscess
            iv. Uretral and renal-pelvic obstruction
        I. Dissecting aneurysm
        J. Intestinal infarction
            i. Mesenteric venous thrombosis
            ii. Mesenteric arterial occlusion due to thrombosis or embolus

GI Bleeding

|One of the most serious and common GI emergencies is GI bleeding. In patients with SCI, it poses a difficult problem both diagnostically and therapeutically. The mortality associated with this entity has been 8% to 10% even with the best management and, in patients with SCI, these figures are higher. Therefore, it is important to have an aggressive and coordinated team approach that makes use of the expertise of nursing, GI medicine, surgery and radiology. Rapid recognition and prompt treatment have critically influenced morbidity and mortality. In the past decade, advances in fiberoptic endoscopy, angiography, and nuclear scanning have led to new dimensions in the diagnosis of previously elusive lesions hemorrhagic gastritis, Mallory-Weiss syndrome, angiodysplasia, etc., and have resulted in the continued emergence of new modalities of therapy. The mortality in acute GI bleeding has decreased due to earlier diagnosis of source of bleeding, new medicines, earlier control of bleeding, and early referral to surgery. The common sources of GI bleeding are listed in Table IV.

|Peptic ulcers are the most common cause of upper GI bleeding (UGIB), accounting for nearly 50% of all cases. Esophageal varices, drug-induced gastritis (alcohol and nonsteroidal anti-inflammatory drugs [NSAIDs]), and stress ulcers are common on patients with SCI.[3, 4, 5]

|Decrease in the incidence of peptic ulcer with eradication of *Helicobacter pylori* and improved healing of ulcers with H_2 receptor antagonists (H_2RA) and proton pump inhibitors (PPI) therapy have considerably reduced the complications of peptic ulcer disease: bleeding, perforations, and pyloro duodenal obstruction.

|Ulcers located high in the lesser curve of the stomach or in the postero inferior wall of the duodenal bulb are more likely to rebleed. Patients with variceal bleed tend to have clinically serious bleeding and rebleeding requiring more transfusions. Mortality in these patients with continued or recurrent bleeding is 50% to 70%. Initial medical therapy consists of intravenous (IV) somatostatin or octreotide. This has largely replaced IV vasopressin. It decreases acid secretion and portal pressure. Endoscopic ligation therapy or sclerotherapy controls variceal bleeding and rebleeding and improves mortality.

|In ulcer bleeding, endoscopic therapy with bipolar electrocoagulation or heater probe controls bleeding and reduces hospital stay, cost, and mortality. Intravenous PPI are commonly used during bleeding. Stress gastritis occurring in intensive care unit patients with respiratory failure, sepsis, shock, jaundice, and thermal burns can cause massive bleeding. Despite aggressive medical, endoscopic, and angiographic therapy, bleeding may persist. Surgical mortality is very high and rebleeding common in these patients. Currently prophylaxis is recommended with IV PPI or H2RA, and PO sucralfate for all seriously ill patients in medical intensive care units. The principles of management of GI bleed constitute resuscitation, diagnosis, and treatment (Table V). Hematemesis is the presenting symptom in 75% of upper GI (UGI) bleeders with the remaining having symptoms of melena without hematemesis. Bright red rectal bleeding more commonly occurs in a lower GI (LGI) bleed. Patients with SCI have a slower colonic and small bowel transit time and may not present with melena until late in the bleed. The clinician must be aware of the motility disturbances in SCI.[6] The pathophysiologic difference between a normal patient with GI bleeding and a patient with SCI are summarized in Table VI.

|As soon as the patient is stable, a specific diagnosis should be made. Depending on the severity and rate of bleeding, endoscopy and/or angiography may be indicated. Generally, the majority of bleeding episodes from both UGI and LGI sources resolve spontaneously. Causes of black stools such as iron or bismuth ingestion should be ruled out. Endoscopy early in the acute bleed is the recommended diagnostic modality and has a higher rate—up to 95%—of providing a diagnosis.

|Frequently, hemorrhoids are the major cause of LGI bleeds. Diverticular disease in SCI is not common and does not constitute a major source of bleeding. Angiodysplasia is now a more prevalent diagnosis in both the SCI and non-SCI population because of better endoscopy and greater awareness by the endoscopist. In patients with SCI, acute LGI bleed is rarely severe and is usually due to hemorrhoids. Initial conservative therapy with subsequent surgery is all that is needed for hemorrhoidal bleeding.

Acute Abdomen
|Acute abdomen refers to sudden and unexpected onset of abdominal pain associated with or without symptoms of nausea, vomiting, abdominal distension, fever, diarrhea or constipation caused by intra-abdominal or extra abdominal causes listed in Table II.[7, 8]

|Colicky pain indicates an obstructive process as in intestinal obstruction, ureteral colic and acute cholecystis. The pain of appendicitis or intra-abdominal abscess is usually gradual in onset, sustained and progressively worse. Ruptured aneurysms or perforated viscus produces a sudden onset of severe excruciating pain. Despite these clear depictions of pain, diagnosis of acute abdomen in patients with SCI is exacting.

|Abdominal pain perception in patients with SCI in general is blunted to varying degrees depending on the level of SCI and completeness of lesion. Visceral pain is vaguely and variously expressed and hardly diagnostic.

|Autonomic symptoms dominate the clinical picture of acute abdominal emergencies in patients with SCI. The higher the spinal lesion, the more pronounced the autonomic symptoms—sweating, pallor, palpitation, tachycardia, hypotension, etc. Patients with lesions below T12 behave clinically like the non-SCI population with regard to acute abdominal emergencies.

|History, physical examination, routine labs and plain films of the abdomen may not help to provide a clear-cut diagnosis. Physical examination is imperfect. Ultrasonagraphy and CT scan are often of great help in the diagnostic evaluation of acute abdomen.

Ileus

|Ileus is a pathophysiologic inhibition of motor activity of the intestines. It is also called adynamic or paralytic ileus. Toxic megacolon is a special form of ileus. Chronic ileus is referred to as pseudo-obstruction. Ogilvie's syndrome is acute idiopathic colonic pseudo-obstruction.

|Paralytic ileus is a frequent disorder in patients with SCI. Its exact incidence is difficult to determine because of different degree and severity of symptoms. Neural, metabolic, humeral, and drug factors play a role in its pathogenesis. Common causes of paralytic ileus in patients with SCI are listed in Table VII.

|Absence of pre-existing pain (abdominal colic) and peristalsis (bowel sounds) are the hallmark of ileus. Patients with SCI may have reflex ileus from infection and have active bowel sounds, air-fluid levels on abdominal films are highly suggestive of mechanical obstruction, but can also occur in adynamic ileus. The problem is resolved with conservative measures, such as nasogastric suction, intravenous hydration, correction of electrolyte abnormalities, and the appropriate treatment of underlying disease. If bowel sounds are present and air-fluid levels are not present, then bowel rest and nasogastric suction may not be needed. Constipation with fecal impaction is a frequently encountered problem in patients with SCI and they usually respond to medical management with hydration, laxatives, and enemas.[9] Preventive measures include daily bowel care, stool softeners, and high-fiber diet and/or bulk laxatives (Metamucil, Perdiem).

|Visceral perforation, mechanical bowel obstruction, cholecystitis, and appendicitis are the most common surgical emergencies. Although surgical intervention is necessary to relieve obstruction and prevent bowel infarction, in most cases of partial mechanical obstruction, conservative measures with suction and intravenous fluids may prevent, at least temporarily, operative intervention in about a quarter of the patients, provided that infarction of the bowel is not a threat. This would involve close observation and frequent re-evaluation, particularly in patients with SCI whose abdominal pain and tenderness are difficult to evaluate. SCI does not eliminate causes of ileus secondary to mechanical obstruction and the clinician should maintain vigilance and remember that in SCI there is a paucity of symptoms. Clinical features that may suggest strangulation are: fever, tachycardia, leukocytosis, shock, hypothermia, and bloody diarrhea. Intestinal obstruction associated with an acute exacerbation of regional enteritis is always best treated conservatively. In recurrent intestinal obstruction from adhesions, repeat operations should be avoided when possible.

|With a better understanding of the pathophysiology of intestinal obstruction and with supportive treatment via parenteral alimentation and antibiotics, and with lysis of surgical adhesions from previous surgery, infections, or trauma, mortality has declined from 60% to less than 5%.

The Major Causes of Mechanical Obstructions in SCI

I. Adhesions from previous surgery, infections, or trauma

II. Abscesses

III. Volvulus (gastric, cecal, sigmoid, midgut)

IV. Neoplasms (adenocarcinoma, lymphoma, carcinoid tumor)

V. Strictures

VI. Pyloroduodenal obstruction

VII. Mesenteric infarction secondary to arterial or venous occlusion

VIII. Strangulated hernia: external or internal

IX. Fecal impaction

X. Barium impaction

|Prior to conclusion, discussion should be given to cholecystitis and pancreatitis. Acute cholecystitis, although infrequent, must be thought of in patients with SCI who have abdominal symptoms. Nuclear scans of bilary function and hepatobiliary scintography, which do not visualize cystic duct, are consistent with acute inflammation of the gallbladder with accuracy of 90%. Prompt surgery is recommended in acute obstructive or fulminant cholecystitis.

|In chronic cholecystitis with gallstones, elective cholecystectomy is the preferred treatment.[10,11,12] Endoscopic surgery is the procedure of choice with minimal risk and rapid recovery. In patients with SCI, endoscopic surgery is recommended in uncomplicated patients who have not had previous abdominal surgery.

|The most common etiology of pancreatitis is acute and chronic alcohol use. The specific mechanism is still debatable. Treatment is conservative and supportive to relieve continued stimulation of the pancreas. The other causes of pancreatitis must not be overlooked—cholelithiasis, peptic ulcer perforation, trauma, surgery, drugs, hypotensive shock, hyperlipidemia, and hyperparathyroidism. In the non-resolving case, ultrasound/CT scan of abdomen must be done to look for pseudocyst or abscess and referral to surgery may be necessary.

|Lastly, one should not overlook the common GI symptoms of nausea and vomiting that may mimic an acute abdomen and may be due to psychogenic vomiting and iatrogenic reactions to drugs or drug withdrawal. Nausea in the patient on dialysis and in end-stage renal disease is not uncommon. GI symptoms may overshadow symptoms of genitourinary infection or renal failure.

Conclusion

|Some of the acute abdominal emergencies have been touched upon, with some emphasis on how they differ from the non-SCI population. Clinical intuition plays a major role in an accurate diagnosis. The surgeon should be alerted and consulted early in all acute abdominal emergencies and the SCI physician always must be alert to varied symptoms that may relate in intra-abdominal pathology. It must be always kept in the clinician's mind that the normal pattern of symptoms of GI emergencies may not be present or may be altered in SCI. The expediency and skill with which an accurate diagnosis is established and appropriate therapy instituted will dictate the outcome.

Table I **Axioms of Spinal Cord Medicine**

I.	The acute GI emergencies in stable patients with SCI are no different from those in the general population except their manifestations are obscure and characterized by paucity of signs and symptoms.
	The higher the level of spinal lesion, the more difficult the diagnosis.
II.	Patient with lesions below T12 should pose no diagnostic dilemma.
	In general, because of the paucity of signs and symptoms, more X-ray studies and diagnostic scans are used and there is a certain delay in diagnosis.
III.	Fever is an important symptom and often signifies renal, retroperitoneal, intraperitoneal, or visceral inflammation and is often accompanied by abdominal distension, nausea, and/or vomiting.
	Referred pain may be an important clue to the diagnosis. Pain of acute cholecystitis radiates to the right shoulder and that of perforated or penetrating gastric/duodenal ulcer may radiate to the left shoulder.
IV.	High index of suspicion Clinical intuition and acumen Detailed history Meticulous examination Go a long way in arriving at a diagnosis. Repeat examinations and close follow-up Appropriate lab and X-ray studies Pertinent consultations

Table II **Acute Abdominal Emergencies in Stable Patients With SCI**

I. Acute GI hemorrhage
II. Acute abdomen
    A. Paralytic ileus
    B. Constipation/obstipation/fecal impaction
    C. Inflammatory conditions
        i. Acute appendicitis
        ii. Acute pancreatitis
        iii. Acute cholecystitis
        iv. Diverticulitis (Diverticulosis is uncommon in patients with SCI)
    D. Intestinal obstruction
        i. Pyloroduodenal
        ii. Small bowel obstruction
        iii. Large bowel obstruction, especially volvulus
        iv. Intestinal obstruction due to strangulated hernia
    E. Hollow viscus perforation
        i. In peptic ulcer disease, inflammatory bowel disease,
          diverticulitis, appendicitis, blunt trauma, and tumor.
    F. Vascular disease
        i. Dissecting aneurysm and abdominal aortic aneurysmal leak
        ii. Mesenteric thrombosis or insufficiency (ischemic bowel disease)
    G. Miscellaneous
        i. Abdominal trauma
        ii. Acute gastric dilatation
        iii. Inflammatory bowel disease with toxic megacolon

Table III **Differences Between Somatic and Visceral Pain**

	Somatic Pain	Visceral Pain
	Precisely localized at disease site	Ill-defined and poorly localized. Often pain is referred to midline (reflecting embryonic derivation of the gut).
Source of pain	Parietal peritoneum	Hollow viscera
Characteristics of pain	Sharp, jabbing pain; sudden onset and of short duration	Cramping, colicky, sickening, or dull aching pain—difficult for the patient to characterize. Lasts longer.
Tenderness of abdomen to palpation	Present, pain gets worse on palpation	Abdominal tenderness absent. There may be actual relief of pain by pressure on a distended gut.
Autonomic symptoms	Usually absent	Usually present. Palpitation, pallor, nausea or sweating often occurs concomitantly.
Tissue damage	Implies potential or actual tissue damage.	May be just a simulation without any real tissue damage.
Pain receptors	Somatic receptors in parietal peritoneum.	Autonomic afferents within the wall of viscus

Table IV **Major Causes of GI Hemorrhage in Patients With SCI**

I. Upper GI Bleeding
    A. Peptic ulcer disease
        i. Duodenal ulcer
        ii. Gastric ulcer
        iii. Esophageal ulcer
    B. Gastritis — Gastric erosions
        i. NSAIDs
        ii. Alcoholic hemorrhagic gastritis
    C. Stress gastritis — Stress ulcers (cushing or curling)
    D. Varices
    E. Mallory Weiss tear
    F. Aorto-enteric fistula
    G. Neoplasms
    H. Angiodysplasia
    I. Uremia
    J. Coagulopathies
    K. Others

II. Lower GI Bleeding in Patients With SCI
    A. Hemorrhoids
    B. Diverticular disease of the colon is an uncommon cause of bleeding (only a few instances of diverticular disease noted in patients with SCI in the past 20 years)
    C. Cancers and polyps
    D. Inflammatory bowel disease
    E. Ischemic colitis
    F. Radiation colitis
    G. Others

Table V **GI Bleeding Management**

I. Resuscitation and monitoring of patient:
    A. Quick evaluation (may require nasogastric intubation) to confirm upper GI bleeding.
    B. Establish IV line
        i. draw blood for appropriate lab studies.
        ii. type and cross-match blood.
        iii. start IV with saline, Ringer's lactate.
    C. Flowsheet depicting the following
        i. Clinical
            a. mental status
            b. pulse
            c. gastric aspirate
            d. urine output
            e. accurate intake and output
        ii. Lab Tests
            a. HgB/Hct
            b. PT/PTT
            c. electrolytes
    D. A thorough history and physical examination with emphasis on medication (aspirin, anticoagulants, NSAIDs, steroids) and cutaneous manifestations of GI disease.
II. Definitive diagnosis: upper endoscopy, colonoscopy, angiography, exploratory surgery if warranted.

Table VI **Clinical Features in GI Bleeding**

Patient With Normal Neuraxis	Patients With SCI
I. Disease entities commonly associated with GI bleeding have a characteristic pain pattern.	Pain pattern absent, altered, or blunted.
II. Pathophysiologic responses: hypotension dizziness tachycardia shock	Pathophysiologic responses in patients with SCI may not be appropriate because they are wheelchair- and bed-bound and because of autonomic vasomotor dysfunction. Patients with SCI basically maintain a low blood pressure and are prone to postural hypotension; hence, there is difficulty in the recognition and appreciation of cardiovascular responses to GI bleeding.
III. Melena	Patients may not notice the color of their stools—the physician has to depend on the nurse, bowel care person, or aide.
IV. Hematemesis is a common manifestation of GI bleeding in 80% to 90% of cases.	Hematemesis is not that common, especially in patients with high quadriplegia.
V. Occult bleeding leads to well-compensated anemia.	Anemia due to other causes is so common that occult GI bleeding as a cause may be overlooked.

Table VII **Common Causes of Ileus in Patients With SCI**

Extra-Abdominal Causes	Intra-Abdominal Causes

I. Drugs:
  A. Anticholinergics
  B. Opiates
II. Metabolic Causes:
  A. Electrolyte imbalance:
    i. Hypokalemia
    ii. Hypomagnesemia
  B. Diabetic ketoacidosis
III. Basal pneumonia
IV. Pulmonary embolism
V. Myocardial infarction
VI. Gram-negative sepsis
	I. Renal colic
	II. Pyelonephritis, cystitis
	III. Perinephric abscess
	IV. Retroperitoneal hemorrhage
	V. Retroperitoneal abscess
	VI. Peritonitis
	VII. Cholecystitis
	VIII. Pancreatitis
	IX. Appendicitis
	X. Infectious enteritis
	XI. Perforated viscus
	XII. Strangulation obstruction
	XIII. Unresolved mechanical obstruction (such as fecal impaction)
	XIV. Post laparotomy

References

1. Wood JD, Alpers DH, Andrews PL. Fundamentals of neurogastroenterology. *Gut* 1999;45 (Suppl 2): II6-II16. Review.

2. Webaurn RB, Pearse AGE, Polalk JM, et al. The APUD cells of the alimentary tract in health and disease. *Med Clin North Am* 1974;58:1359.

3. Soderstrom CA, Ducker TB. Increased susceptibility of patients with cervical cord lesions to peptic gastrointestinal complications. *J Trauma* 1985;25:1030-1038.

4. Kiwerski J. Bleeding from the alimentary canal during the management of spinal cord injury patients. *Paraplegia* 1986;24:92-96.

5. Gore RM, Mintzer RA, Calenoff L. Gastrointestinal complication of spinal cord injury. *Spine* 1981;6:538-544.

6. Glick ME, Meshkinpour H, Haldemann S, et al. Colonic dysfunction in patients with thoracic spinal cord injury. *Gastroenterology* 1987;92:966-968.

7. Juler GL, Eltorai IM. The acute abdomen in spinal cord injury patients. *Paraplegia* 1985;23:1118-123.

8. Bar-on Z, Ohry A. The acute abdomen in spinal cord injury individuals. *Paraplegia* 1995;33:704-706.

9. Badiali D, Bracci F, Castellano V, Corazziari E, et al. Sequential treatment of chronic constipation in paraplegic subjects. *Spinal Cord* 1997;35(2):116-120.

10. Apstein MD, Dalecki-Chipperfield K. Spinal cord injury is a risk factor for gallstone disease. *Gastroenterology* 1987;92:1143-1148.

11. Moonka R, Steins SA, Renick WJ, et al. The prevalence and natural history of gallstones in spinal cord injured patients. *J Am Coll Surg* 1999;189:274-281.

12. Moonka R, Steins SA, Eubank EB, et al. The presentation of gallstones and results of biliary surgery in a spinal cord injured population. *Am J Surg* 1999;178:246-250.

Ibrahim M. Eltorai, ° MD;
James G. Jakowatz, MD;
George L. Juler, MD

The |ACUTE ABDOMEN

CHAPTER SIX

|Patients with spinal cord injury (SCI), whether paraplegic or tetraplegic, present challenging problems to the abdominal surgeons when they develop an acute abdomen.

|The problems are due to sensory deficits, unremarkable symptoms and signs, associated pathophysiological changes, such as fecal impaction due to colonic stasis, colosphincteric dyssynergia, adynamic ileus, radicular pains, urinary tract infection (UTI), spasticity, vasomotor changes, especially autonomic hyperreflexia, cardiopulmonary disease, electrolyte imbalances, psychological disturbances, drug use and abuse.

|Taking a careful history and physical examination with laboratory tests should not be delayed even with the least suspicion to avoid higher mortality in this population. The surgical interventions are the same as in individuals without SCI, but a close watch with assessment is needed to avoid post-operative complications.

Introduction

|In the United States, the incidence of SCI is approximately 50 to 55 persons per million.[1-4] Of these, 15 cases die at or close to the onset of trauma due to multiple injuries or high-cord injuries leading to respiratory arrest. Each year approximately 12,000 new injuries are added to the SCI population. Five to 10 cases sustain minor cord or root injuries and about 15 per million or 9,000 to 10,000 cases are admitted to medical centers where they are rehabilitated and need prolonged care. With the decreasing mortality since World War II, and with the increasing longevity almost to that of the general population, there are approximately a quarter million patients with SCI who require continuing, sometimes intense, medicosurgical care. Over 80% are males, with a median age of 25 years. However, the elderly and children are not exempt, the former especially from spondylosis and the latter from road accident and even at birth. The etiological details cannot be presented in this chapter. In addition to traumatic cord dysfunction, there are other non-traumatic causes that lead to the syndrome called "Spinal Man." These may be congenital, iatrogenic, inflammatory, idiopathic, or neoplastic and degenerative diseases. As a result of spinal cord dysfunction, there is a loss of motor and sensory functions, loss of bowel and bladder control, and loss of normal sexual function. The degree of these losses depends on the extent of the cord and/or cauda equina damage and its level. The result is "Spinal Man," whether paraplegic or quadriplegic, complete, or incomplete. The popular term "paraplegic" may apply at any level.

Pathophysiology

|The following changes are of importance to remember when examining a patient with paraplegia:

   I. Disruption of somatic sensation. This may be complete in complete cord transection or incomplete especially in blunt cord trauma, ischemic myelopathy, and other causes.[5]

   II. Visceral sensation may be less affected than the somatic one and this may be explained by:

   A. Visceral sensory fibers ascending several levels along the autonomic ganglia before entering the cord thus bypassing the damaged cord segments.

   B. Some visceral fibers escaping damage in the cord.

   C. Some visceral afferents traveling through the phrenic and possibly vagus nerves.

III. Loss of voluntary function of the skeletal muscles. In the stage of spinal shock, it is flaccid paralysis. This will remain in the muscles innervated by the damaged segments at the level of injury, below that level, the muscles will regain reflex activity and become spastic except in those cases of infarcted cord or with longitudinal damage of the cord. This is what Comarr calls "The Law of the Spinal Cord."[6] Spasticity of the abdominal muscles may mimic an acute abdomen or may mask it.

IV. Vasomotor changes.[7]

    A. Postural hypotension may lead to syncope with pallor and sometimes nausea associated with tachycardia. This may be misleading in diagnosis of acute abdomen.

    B. Autonomic dysreflexia is an acute syndrome of a massive disordered autonomic response to a specific stimulus in patients with high SCI located at or above T6.[8-11] Although this syndrome occurs in over 83% of such a group of patients, it is often not recognized or is misdiagnosed by physicians unfamiliar with patients with SCI. The condition may be fatal if not recognized and managed properly, mostly due to cerebral hemorrhage.[12] The causative stimuli are usually distended or spastic bladder, rectal distension or impaction, acute abdominal conditions, urinary calculi, sigmoidoscopy, cystoscopy, manipulations in the gastrointestinal (GI) or genitourinary (GU) tracts, somatic stimuli from fractures, decubiti, etc. As a result of these stimuli reaching the isolated cord, reflex sympathetic stimuli through the lateral horns of the spinal cord cause severe splanchnic and peripheral vasoconstriction and lead to severe hypertension. Normally the baroreceptors are stimulated and they inhibit both the vagus and the vasomotor center. In SCI, vasoconstriction persists and the vagal tone is increased so that the hypertension is generally accompanied by bradycardia. This syndrome is very important as it may mimic acute abdominal conditions or may be a manifestation of an acute abdomen. (See chapter 1.)

V. Pseudomotor function and thermoregulation are disturbed. Patients with SCI may be poikilothermic, developing hypothermia in cold environments and hyperthermia in hot environments due to interruption of the mechanisms of thermoregulation.[14] This may be confusing in the diagnosis of acute abdomen. (See Chapter 21.)

VI. GI changes.[13,14]

    A. In the stage of spinal shock, there is GI atony with gastric dilation and intestinal stasis.

    B. Upon recovery, the patients have a tendency to develop stress ulcers especially if they have a history of ulcers. Bleeding may be an emergency in some cases. In chronic cases, acute and chronic dilation may be noticed due to gastric dysmotility, pyloric spasm, and aerophagia as evidenced by prolonged transit time. *Helicobacter pylori* infection is not uncommon in chronic cases.

    C. Small bowel. Apart from paralytic ileus in the acute stage, no specific pathophysiology was proven in the small bowel. However, there may be small intestinal pseudo-obstruction noted clinically and radiographically. Patients with SCI above the splanchnic outlet, i.e., above T7, may show dilation with fluid levels. Small bowel gas shadows may be due to bowel obstruction from fecal impaction or colonic dysmotility. Adynamic ileus has been noticed in patients with injuries above T7 as a manifestation of sympathetic inhibitory reflexes.

    D. Colon. Fecal impaction due to inadequate propulsion and increased rectal sphincter tone (recto-anal dyssynergia) lead to distension. This will progress eventually to megasigmoid and megacolon, which aggravate the stasis, especially in lumbosacral lesions. Diverticulosis and/or volvulus may eventually ensue in some cases. On the other hand, the impacted bowel may lead to overflow diarrhea or diarrhea paradoxa.14 Hemorrhoids and/or anal fissures develop in some patients, especially those with cauda equina lesion.

    E. Gallbladder. There is a tendency to believe that patients with SCI have an independent risk factor for cholelithiasis, especially patients with a level above T7. Ultrasonic studies showed that patients with a level above T7 had resting volume and ejection fraction significantly lower than those of the controls but the emptying time and residual volume were normal. Because of the difficulty in the physical signs, one should suspect gallbladder disease based on symptoms such as nausea, vomiting, indigestion, flatulence, hyperhidrosis, and dysreflexia in absence of other causes. Ultrasound examination should be done even if very doubtful.

F. Pancreas. No specific pathology in the pancreas was detected as a result of cord injury except with direct trauma. However, the presence of acute and chronic pancreatitis is mostly associated with alcoholism and gallbladder disease.

|Pain in SCI has been classified into five types: peripheral, central, visceral, mechanic, and psychic.[8] We are more concerned with the visceral type although other types may be confusing in diagnosis of acute abdomen, e.g., radicular pain may simulate gallbladder or appendicular disease. Visceral pain from abdominal pathology is perhaps conducted along the sympathetic fibers and sacral parasympathetic fibers in pelvic pathology. Participation of the vagus is doubtful. Another kind of pain is the referred pain mostly from the ulcer perforation, i.e., to the shoulder or superclavicular area. Patients with injury level below T12 will behave like others with normal neuraxis.

Surgical Diagnosis of Acute Abdomen [15-19]

|The aforementioned pathophysiologic changes make early recognition, diagnosis, and management of the acute abdomen in patients with SCI very difficult. It mandates that the physicians taking care of them reduce the mortality and morbidity by avoiding delay in surgical intervention. It is interesting to mention that by the turn of the last century, the mortality of acute abdominal conditions in patients with SCI ranged from 50% to 80% according to a report by Burrell in a Boston hospital.[20] At the end of World War II, mortality fell to 27%. In the 1950s it dropped to 10% and after that to 5%, and in our series, previously reported, it was 4.75%. It is important that physicians take a full history of the patient, past and present. The symptoms have to be carefully analyzed. A paraplegist would participate with the surgeon and the urologist.

Symptomatology

|Anorexia is one of the earliest symptoms of acute abdomen. Frequently, the patient states: "There is something wrong with my abdomen, I don't feel well." Nausea and vomiting are later manifestations, especially in incomplete lesions. Referred pain, specifically to the shoulder, is a manifestation of viscus perforation of a peptic ulcer. Increased spasticity of abdominal muscles is noted and may even be seen in the extremities.

Hyperhydrosis

|Increasing reflex spinal sweating is frequently associated with visceral inflammation and bowel distension. Because of sympathetic overlap, the level of sweating may be lower or higher than the level of anesthesia. Patients with lesions below the splanchnic outflow do not show reflex sweating. Autonomic dysreflexia, manifested by pounding headache and sudden elevation of the blood pressure, systolic and diastolic, usually with bradycardia and sometimes tachycardia, is a frequent manifestation of high lesions.

|Abdominal distension is a common finding in patients with SCI. It is of gradual onset and progressive. However, if it is acute onset and progressive, the distension is likely to be abnormal.

Physical Signs

General examination: Pyrexia, tachycardia, hypertension, hypotension, sweating, and sick appearance all may appear in patients with chronic SCI without an acute abdomen. These patients, as mentioned previously, may have environmental pyrexia and hyperhydrosis above the level of injury. Also patients with quadriplegia may experience hypertension and autonomic dysreflexia. Therefore, from the beginning, one should not rush to a conclusion. In addition, pain may be of neurogenic or psychogenic origin. However, the presence of one or more of these signs is significant.

Local examination: Assessment of the acute abdomen in patients with SCI is rather difficult for the general surgeon who does not deal with this population on a frequent basis. The signs are:

I. Abdominal musculature guarding. Although this is an important sign in normal individuals, it might be misleading in patients with SCI except in lumbrosacral or cauda injuries. Spasticity is generally intermittent, whereas abdominal guarding from an inflamed viscus may be persistent and change from tonic to clonic. A change of extremity spasticity from extension to flexion is significant.

II. Tenderness may not be elicited but, if it is present, it usually indicates perforated viscus. In these cases there is invariably shoulder pain. Localized tenderness, when present and rebound, usually indicates an inflamed or perforated viscus.

III. Distension of the abdomen is common in patients with SCI due to constipation, fecal impaction, intestinal fermentation, etc. If this appears suddenly and progresses, then it is important and may indicate acute abdomen.

IV. Bowel sounds are rarely significant but, when they have been hyperactive and suddenly become silent, a bowel obstruction is a possibility. It is always important to remember a dynamic ileus in the setting of chronic SCI. Hypermobility of the bowel may be correlated with the stage of spinal shock with the use of spasmolytics for bladder spasms (Ditropan, Pro-Banthine, calcium channel blockers).

V. Abdominal tympany to percussion usually represents flatulence or a chronically distended colon in the majority of patients. Dullness to percussion over the liver may be obliterated in visceral perforation. Detection of frank peritonitis may be difficult.

VI. Other signs, e.g., rebound tenderness (Blumberg's sign), pain on coughing, Rosving's sign, Murphy's sign, if detected, may be helpful but are not entirely dependable. Findings already reported on 42 cases have been thoroughly reviewed.[17] Seven additional cases from hospital records may be edited as examples of delayed diagnosis:

   A. A 53-year-old male with quadriplegia developed cecal volvulus, which was diagnosed late. Despite treatment with a right hemicolectomy, the patient succumbed in the postoperative period.

   B. A 74-year-old male with quadriplegia, ventilator-dependent, developed sigmoid volvulus, not diagnosed in time. He had a sigmoid colectomy and Meckel's diverticulectomy, but succumbed after a stormy postoperative course.

   C. A 69-year-old male with quadriplegia developed massive GI bleeding from gastric ulcers, had a subtotal gastrectomy and also succumbed after a stormy postoperative course.

   D. A 66-year-old with paraplegia, T4, presented with cholelithiasis, had an open cholecystectomy, and had respiratory failure necessitating ventilator assistance. Fortunately, he eventually recovered.

   E. A 69-year-old with paraplegia, T6, presented with abdominal cramps and was found to have a pulmonary carcinoid with metastasis to the liver and the bone. He succumbed later without intervention.

   F. A 66-year-old with paraplegia presenting UTI due to renal stone developed a urinoma, which was drained but he succumbed from ARDS. This is a very rare example of stone ulceration through the kidney pelvis.

Laboratory Tests

Urine examination: For pyuria and bacteriuria may be diagnostic of UTI. However, the majority of patients with SCI carry some pus cells and bacteria, especially when they have an indwelling catheter. This may be misleading and may divert the attention from an acute abdomen with serious consequences.

Blood studies:

I. Blood picture. High white count is an evidence of suppuration, somewhere, possibly an acute abdomen or acute kidney infection. A shift to the left is of significance but is not quite marked. It is important to know that patients with SCI tend to have a lower white count than the average individual.

II. Blood chemistry—bilirubin, pancreatic enzymes, electrolytes, etc.—are important for differential diagnosis.

Acute abdominal series: This should be swiftly ordered. Patients with perforation of the viscus will have free air within the peritoneal cavity. Cholelithiasis, urolithiasis, fluid levels, fecaliths, or fecalomas may be detected.

Chest X-rays: X-rays will rule out pulmonary disease that might give abdominal symptoms, especially with pulmonary embolism and pleurisy. Upright chest X-rays will add to the detection of free air.

Contrast radiography: Upper GI series if needed; IVP or cystography. If urinary tract disease or bladder perforation is suspected, cystography is indicated. Gastrograffin enema or water-soluble enema may be needed to rule out volvulus or other diseases. Computer-aided tomography (CT) scan with contrast is most helpful in ambiguous cases. This test should be used early in the patient's symptoms and as the first diagnostic intervention. Diagnostic accuracy with CT scanning has greatly improved over the last 5 years and is often better in the diagnosis of appendicitis, ruptured viscus, diverticulitis, retroperitoneal abscess, retroperitoneal fluid/hematoma, pneumatosis intestinalis, bowel obstruction, etc. Other tests, such as angiography, may be needed if ischemic bowel disease or leaking aneurysms are suspected. MRI may be needed in difficult cases. However, it is very important to request a CT scan with contrast from the beginning to reach and early diagnosis.

Ultrasonography:[21]

I. Cholesystosonography is diagnostic of acute cholecystitis, calculous or noncalculous, emphysematous gallbladder, gangrene, and perforation of the gallbladder and cholelithiasis.

II. Renal sonography may be diagnostic of kidney obstruction and/or calculi.

III. Ultrasonography of the appendix may show a fecolith, wall thickness, luminar dilation, or perforation. It is advisable to perform pansonography of the abdomen and pelvis in these patients.

IV. In the female patient, ectopic pregnancy, uterine, or adnexal pathology may be diagnosed by this test.

Isotope studies:

I. Gallium- or indium-labeled white blood cell scans may be used in less emergent conditions when sonography is not decisive.

Endoscopic diagnosis:

I. Cystoscopy may be used for UTI.

II. Proctosigmoidoscopy may be used for lower bowel problems.

III. Upper GI endoscopy may be diagnostic for suspected gastric or duodenal lesions.

IV. Laparoscopy may be diagnostic and therapeutic in rare cases.

|In abdominal emergencies, we found a CT scan with contrast most helpful as the first and most important diagnostic test.

Management

|Surgical interventions do not differ from those of patients with normal neuraxis. However, there are certain differences:

I. Prompt intervention when the diagnosis is made. Mortality may be higher in this group, especially the elderly, as noted in the cases mentioned previously.

II. Anesthesia. These patients are anesthetic due to their injury but spinal anesthesia is a valuable means to avoid dysreflexia. General anesthesia may be required.

III. Meticulous parietal wall closure to avoid dehiscence due to postoperative distension and/or spasm.

IV. Postoperative complications are higher: sepsis, pulmonary complications especially, atelectasis, decubiti, paralytic ileus, and deep vein thrombosis. These are preventable in most cases.

V. Fluid and electrolyte balance should be maintained.

VI. Antibiotic therapy is essential.

Conclusion

I. Patients with paraplegia or quadriplegia constitute a different group of patients due to various pathophysiological changes that occur as a result of SCI. Sensory loss is a primary reason for delay in diagnosis. Associated problems, such as GU infections, fecal impaction, adynamic ileus, radicular or spinal cord pain, drug and alcohol use, psychological disturbances, and cardiorespiratory disease may complicate the picture and lead to misdiagnosis. This delays intervention in acute abdominal conditions and may lead to an unnecessary surgery.

II. The various degrees of cord injury and the different levels do not give a typical picture to spot the diagnosis.

III. Autonomic dysreflexia in patients paralyzed at T6 or above may complicate the picture and, if not managed properly, may lead to cerebral hemorrhage and vascular collapse. The symptoms and signs are not typical and may seem trivial but should not be overlooked.

IV. Careful history, clinical examination, laboratory tests, early CT scanning should be promptly ordered and when diagnosis is made, early intervention is necessary to avoid high mortality.

V. Surgical intervention follows the standard techniques with precautions to avoid postoperative morbidity and mortality.

VI. Physicians not familiar with these patients should consult with SCI specialists.

References

1. Kraus JF, Foranti CE, Riggins RS, et al. Incidence of traumatic spinal cord lesions. *J Chr Dis* 1975;28:471-492.

2. Griffin MR, O'Falon WM, Opitz JL, Turland LT. Mortality, survival and prevalence: traumatic spinal cord injury in Olmstead County, Minnesota 1935-1981. *J Chr Dis* 1985;38(8):643-653.

3. Kraus JF, Foranti CE, Borhani NO, Riggins RS. Survival with an acute spinal cord injury. *J Chr Dis* 1979;32:269-283.

4. Bracken MB, Freeman DH, Hellenbrand K. Incidence of acute traumatic hospitalized spinal cord injury in the United States 1970-1977. *Am J Ep* 1981;113(6):615-622.

5. Hoen TI, Cooper IS. Acute abdominal emergencies in paraplegics. *Am J Surg* 1948;75:19-24.

6. Guttmann L. Clinical aspects of spinal cord injuries. In: Guttmann L. (Ed). *Spinal Cord Injuries. Comprehensive Management and Research.* 1973, Blackwell Scientific Publications: Oxford; pp.259-261.

7. Guttmann L. *Spinal cord injuries comprehensive management and research.* Blackwell, Oxford, 1976:305-330.

8. Donovan WH, Dimitrijevic MR, Dahm L, Dimitrijevic M. Neurophysical approaches to chronic pain following spinal cord injury. *Paraplegia* 1982;20:135-146.

9. Comarr AE. Neurology of spinal cord injured patients. *Seminars in Urology* 1992;10(2):74-82.

10. Trop CS, Bennett CJ. The evaluation of autonomic dysreflexia. *Seminars in Urology* 1992;10(2):95-101.

11. Cole JD. The paraphysiology of the autonomic nervous system in spinal cord injury. In: Illis LS. (Ed). *Spinal Cord Dysfunction Assessment.* Oxford University Press: Oxford 1988.

12. Calachis SC. Autonomic hyperreflexia with spinal cord injury. *J Am Para Soc* 1992:15(3):171-186.

13. Eltorai I, Kim R, Vulpe M, et al. Fatal cerebral hemorrhage due to autonomic dysreflexia in a tetraplegic patient: case report and review. *Paraplegia* 1992;30:355-360.

14. Cosman BD, Stone IM, Perkash I. Gastrointestinal complications of chronic spinal cord injury. *J Am Para Soc* 1991;14(4):175-181.

15. Guttmann L. *Spinal cord injuries comprehensive management and research: Disturbances of internal function*. Blackwell, Oxford, 1976:458-473.

16. Burrell cited by: Neumayer LA, Bull DA, Mahr JD, Putnam CW. The acutely affected abdomen in paraplegic spinal cord injury patients. *Ann Surg* 1990;212(5):561-566.

17. Juler GL, Eltorai IM. The acute abdomen in spinal cord injury patients. *Paraplegia* 1985;23:118-123.

18. Charney KJ, Juler GL, Comarr AE. General surgery problems in patients with spinal cord injury. *Arch Surg* 1975;110:1083-1088.

19. Juler GL. Acute abdominal emergencies in patients with spinal cord lesions. *J Am Para Soc* 1979;2:1-5.

20. Lang FC. Ultrasonography of the acute abdomen. *Radiologic clinics of North America*. 1992; 30(2):389-404.

* Part of this chapter was presented to the XXVIII World Congress of the International College of Surgeons Cairo-Egypt Nov 16-21, 1992 Monduzzi Editore. Bologna, Italy

|UROLOGIC
Regina M. Hovey, MD

Emergencies in Patients With SCI

CHAPTER SEVEN ▆▆▆▆▆▆▆▆▆▆▆

|Preservation of renal function is the primary goal in the urologic management of patients with spinal cord injuries (SCI). With closer urologic surveillance and improvement in long-term urologic management, renal failure is no longer the leading cause of death in this population.[1,2] Although emphasis is placed on preventive care, urologic emergencies are still common. Because of impaired sensation, the clinical presentation may be different than in a patient who is neurologically intact. The following is a discussion of the most common urologic emergencies in patients with SCI.

Urinary Tract Infection (UTI) and Urosepsis
|Most patients with SCI and neurogenic bladder will have chronic colonization of the urine with bacteria. Treatment for asymptomatic bacteriuria is not recommended. Patients with symptomatic UTI (fevers, chills, dysuria, significant pyuria, worsening bladder spasms) should be treated with appropriate antibiotics. Other sources for infection (lungs, wounds, etc.) should be ruled out as well.

|In patients with a symptomatic UTI or urosepsis, renal imaging should be obtained to rule out urinary obstruction or stones. Appropriate imaging studies include a renal/bladder ultrasound and kidney, ureter, and bladder (KUB) or a computer-aided tomography (CT) scan of the abdomen and pelvis. Intravenous pyelography (IVP) may be necessary to further delineate the anatomy.

|Patients with urosepsis require prompt attention. The patient should be started on broad spectrum antibiotics, and resuscitated with intravenous fluids and pressors if necessary. If urinary obstruction is present, relief of the obstruction is necessary using endoscopic or percutaneous techniques.

Urinary Obstruction

|Urinary obstruction can occur at several different levels: kidney, ureter, bladder, and urethra. The diagnosis can be made by routine screening of the upper tracts in an asymptomatic patient, or by imaging performed in a patient with a symptomatic UTI or urosepsis. Hydronephrosis and hydroureter are often present in urinary obstruction, but may be chronic and are not diagnostic. A diuretic renal scan may be necessary to diagnose obstruction in a patient with a chronically dilated upper urinary tract.

|Urinary obstruction at the level of the bladder or urethra can be temporarily treated by placement of a Foley catheter or a suprapubic catheter if a Foley catheter cannot be passed. Kidney and ureteral obstruction can be initially managed by endoscopic placement of a ureteral stent or by placement of a percutaneous nephrostomy tube. A percutaneous nephrostomy tube should be placed if attempted endoscopic stent placement is unsuccessful or if the patient has a symptomatic urinary infection (fever, chills, significant pyuria, or urosepsis). Attempts at endoscopic manipulation in a patient with an obstructed and infected urinary tract may lead to bacteremia and urosepsis.

|The most common cause of upper tract obstruction in patients with SCI is urinary stones. The overall incidence of renal stones is 14.8% in patients with SCI.[3] Because of impaired sensation, an obstructing stone may not present with renal colic as it will in a patient who is neurologically intact. An obstructing stone should be managed by initial placement of a ureteral stent or percutaneous nephrostomy tube, and subsequent removal of the stone. A non-obstructing stone can be managed definitively on a more elective basis.

Renal Abscess and Perirenal Abscess

|Renal and perirenal abscesses usually arise as complications of pyelonephritis or urinary stones. A renal abscess is located within the renal parenchyma and a perirenal abscess is located in the surrounding fatty tissue within Gerota's fascia. Patients typically present with fevers, chills, leukocytosis, and flank pain. Because of impaired sensation, a patient with SCI may present only with fever or sepsis. An abdominal or flank mass may be palpable. The clinical course can be insidious in onset. The diagnosis can be made with CT or ultrasonography; however, CT is the imaging modality of choice.

|Renal and perirenal abscesses represent serious problems that can have high mortality rates, especially when treatment is delayed. Patients should be started immediately on broad-spectrum antibiotics. Although antibiotics alone can cure a certain percentage of renal abscesses, most cases of renal abscess and all cases of perirenal abscess require drainage. Successful drainage can be performed percutaneously in most cases under CT or ultrasound guidance. If percutaneous drainage fails, the next step is open surgical drainage. If the kidney is poorly functioning, nephrectomy can be performed. Prompt initiation of antibiotic therapy and appropriate drainage will decrease the morbidity and mortality associated with renal and perirenal abscesses.

Priapism

|Priapism is a prolonged erection not related to sexual desire and constitutes a urologic emergency. It is most commonly caused by intracavernosal injection of vasoactive drugs used to treat impotence. In the absence of vascular disease, patients with SCI are more prone to priapism than the general population.[4-6] Other causes of priapism include alcohol and drug abuse, neoplasm, sickle cell disease, trauma, and drugs that affect the nervous system. Patients who are started on intracavernosal injection therapy to treat impotence should be counseled regarding the signs of priapism. Any patient who has an erection that lasts longer than 2 hours should call the urologist. Any patient who has an erection lasting longer than 3 hours should come to the urology clinic or to the emergency room after hours. Priapism can result in permanent impotence in up to 50% of cases, especially if treatment is delayed.[7]

|Treatment includes aspiration of blood through a needle placed in the corpora cavernosa. If the erection resolves, the corpora can be irrigated with sterile saline. If the erection persists, inject the corpora cavernosa with epinephrine (10 to 20 mg in 1 ml of normal saline) or phenylephrine (100 to 200 mg in 1 ml of normal saline). Blood pressure must be monitored closely as a transient rise in blood pressure can occur. Surgical measures may be required if all other treatments fail. Surgical options include creation of a fistula between the corpus cavernosum and the glans penis (Winter procedure) or creation of a shunt between the corpus spongiosum and the cavernosum (Quackles procedure).

Hematuria

|The most common causes of hematuria are infection, stones, trauma, prostatic enlargement, and cancer. Gross hematuria is a urologic emergency and requires immediate attention. Urine culture should be sent and the patient should be started on appropriate antibiotics. A Foley catheter should be gently passed if there is not already one in place. The bladder should be hand irrigated free of any clots. If the catheter is at risk of clotting off, continuous bladder irrigation should be initiated through a 3-way Foley catheter. If bleeding persists, a cystoscopy should be performed to further diagnose the source of bleeding. Any bleeding areas should be resected or fulgurated as necessary. Diffuse, persistent bleeding from the bladder mucosa may require intravesical instillation of alum, silver nitrate, or formalin. Renal imaging (renal ultrasound and KUB, CT, or IVP) should be obtained to evaluate for an upper tract cause of the hematuria.

Epididymitis/Orchitis

|Epididymitis and orchitis are common in patients with SCI, especially in the presence of a chronic Foley catheter. There is a 100% incidence of significant bacteriuria (>100,000 organisms/mL) in patients with long-term indwelling catheters.[8] Foley catheters can cause blockage of the ejaculatory ducts with retrograde spread of urethral bacteria, leading to epididymitis and orchitis. The typical presentation is enlargement and induration of the testicle and/or epididymis. Pain may be present if sensation is intact. The overlying scrotal skin may be erythematous or fixed to the testicle. Treatment consists of appropriate antibiotics based on urine culture results and elevation of the testicle. Intravenous antibiotics may be necessary for severe cases. For persistent or severe cases, especially if there is scrotal skin involvement, a scrotal ultrasound should be performed to rule out an abscess. If an abscess is present, surgical drainage is indicated and an orchiectomy may need to be performed. A suprapubic catheter should be placed in patients who use long-term Foley catheters and have persistent epididymo-orchitis. A minimum of 4 weeks of antibiotics is required to adequately treat the infection.

Prostatitis/Urethritis

|Patients with SCI are at risk for developing prostatitis and urethritis, especially in the presence of long-term Foley catheterization. Foley catheters can cause blockage of the prostatic ducts, leading to prostatitis. If inadequately treated, acute prostatitis, and urethritis can lead to prostatic abscess and periurethral abscess, respectively. If an abscess is present, drainage will be required. Prostatic abscesses may be drained transrectally under ultrasound guidance, but transurethral resection of the prostate may be necessary for adequate drainage. If a periurethral abscess is present, surgical debridement will be necessary. Typically, extensive urethral involvement is present and a suprapubic catheter should be placed. Antibiotic therapy should be based on culture results and should be administered for a minimum of 4 weeks.

Catheter Malfunction

|Some patients with SCI require chronic indwelling urinary catheters (Foley or suprapubic catheter) for management of neurogenic bladder. Sometimes removal of the catheter can be complicated by failure of the catheter balloon to deflate. Removal of the catheter without proper deflation of the balloon can lead to injury of the bladder or urethra, and every effort must be made to deflate the balloon prior to catheter removal. The assistance of a urologist may be necessary. Catheter failure may be due to mechanical failure, improper use, or extrinsic compression. The side port of the catheter may be obstructed with debris or the balloon may be encrusted with crystals or calculi.[9]

|Injection of a few milliliters of normal saline into the side port may dislodge debris and allow the balloon to deflate.[9] The next option is to cut the side port of the catheter underneath the valve. If the balloon still does not deflate, more saline can be injected into the side port with an angiocatheter. A guidewire may also be passed into the side port in attempt to dislodge debris. If these maneuvers are unsuccessful, more invasive techniques will need to be used.

|Injection of 10 to 15 ml of mineral oil into the side port can be effective in certain cases.[10] If the balloon has not deflated after waiting 30 minutes, an additional 10 ml of mineral oil can be injected. If all other maneuvers fail, the balloon may be punctured transrectally or transvaginally under ultrasound guidance, or the balloon can be hyperinflated to the point of rupture with saline.[9] It is important to inspect the balloon after catheter removal and remove any retained balloon fragments from the bladder cystoscopically.

|Meticulous catheter maintenance will help reduce catheter complications. Only sterile water (not saline) should be used for inflation of catheter balloons and indwelling catheters should be changed every 3 to 4 weeks.

Autonomic Dysreflexia

|Autonomic dysreflexia is a syndrome of massive disordered autonomic discharge in response to afferent visceral stimulation. The clinical features include sweating, headaches, nasal congestion, facial flushing, piloerection, and hypertension. The most common cause of autonomic dysreflexia is noxious stimuli from the bladder.[11] It is important to ensure that the bladder is adequately drained when a patient experiences autonomic dysreflexia.

Conclusion

|Although no longer the leading cause of mortality, urologic complications are still quite common in patients with SCI. Because of impaired sensation, many of these complications can be asymptomatic and the clinical presentation may be different than in a patient who is neurologically intact. Health care providers must have a high index of suspicion and take an aggressive approach in diagnosing and treating urologic problems.

References

1. Geisler WO, Jousse AT, Wynne-Jones M, et al. Survival in traumatic spinal cord injury. *Paraplegia* 1983;21:364.

2. Webb DR, Fitzpatrick JM, O'Flynn JD. A 15-year follow-up of 406 consecutive spinal cord injuries. *Br J Urol* 1984;56:614.

3. Hall MK, Hackler RH, Zampiere TA, et al. Renal calculi in spinal cord injured patient: Association with reflux, bladder stones, and Foley catheter drainage. *Urology* 1986;24:126.

4. Bodner DR, Lindan R, Laffler E, et al. The application of intracavernous injection of vasoactive medications for erection in men with spinal cord injury. *J Urol* 1987;138:310.

5. Sidi AA, Cameron JS, Dykstra DD, et al. Vasoactive intracavernous pharmacotherapy for the treatment of erectile impotence in men with spinal cord injury. *J Urol* 1987;138:539.

6. Lloyd LK, Richard JS. Intracavernous pharmacotherapy for management of erectile dysfunction in spinal cord injury. *Paraplegia* 1989;27:457.

7. Macfarlane MT. *Urology for the house officer*, 2nd ed. Williams and Wilkins: Baltimore, 1995.

8. Warren JW, Tenney JH, Hoopes JM, et al. A prospective study of bacteriuria in patients with chronic indwelling urethral catheters. *J Infect Dis* 1982;146:719.

9. Reigle MD, Sandock DS, Resnick MI. When a Foley catheter won't deflate. *Contemporary Urology* 1996;8:51.

10. Murphy GF, Wood DP Jr. The use of mineral oil to manage the nondeflating Foley catheter. *Urology* 1993;149:89.

11. Lindan R, Joiner B, Freehafer AA, et al. Incidence and clinical features of autonomic dysreflexia in patients with spinal cord injury. *Paraplegia* 1980;18:285.

HYPERGLYCEMIC AND HYPOGLYCEMIC

Emergencies in Patients With SCI

James K. Schmitt, MD; Meena Midha, MD;
Norma D. McKenzie, MD

CHAPTER EIGHT

|Hyperglycemia[1] and hypoglycemia occur with increased frequency in patients with spinal cord disease. Spinal cord injury (SCI), with its protean medical complications, may alter the presentation and outcome of these conditions. However, by combining our knowledge of these problems in ambulatory patients with the special features of SCI, a reasonable approach to these emergencies in patients with SCI may be formulated.

Fuel Homeostasis

|In order to understand disorders of hyperglycemia and hypoglycemia, it is useful to briefly review body fuel homeostasis.[1] Glucose and free fatty acids are the major body fuels. Insulin is the most important hormone in the regulation of glucose and fat metabolism. Insulin inhibits lipolysis in fat tissue and hepatic gluconeogenesis. Following a meal, rising glucose levels stimulate insulin secretion by the pancreatic beta cells, which in turn increases glucose uptake by muscle and returns blood glucose to normal. In the fasting state, insulin is at its lowest level. However, the basal level of insulin continues to inhibit lipolysis and gluconeogenesis. Accelerated lipolysis and gluconeogenesis occur when insulin is absent. Opposing the effects of insulin are counterregulatory hormones glucagon, epinephrine, cortisol and growth hormone, which stimulate glycogenolysis and lipolysis. Of these hormones, glucagon and epinephrine are the most potent. Acute hypoglycemia suppresses endogenous insulin production and stimulates secretion of the counterregulatory hormones, returning the blood glucose level to normal.

Diabetes Mellitus in Patients With SCI

|Duckworth et al[2] found that 56% of patients with SCI had abnormal carbohydrate tolerance when given a standard glucose challenge. Stimulated insulin levels tended to be higher in patients with SCI than in ambulatory patients. Therefore SCI results in insulin resistance and type II, non-insulin-dependent diabetes mellitus. The reasons for the insulin resistance in SCI are increased adiposity, inactivity, and decreased glucose disposal by muscles.[3]

|In contrast to type II diabetes mellitus, patients with type I (insulin-dependent) diabetes have little or no insulin response to a glucose challenge. Although type I diabetes occurs no more frequently in patients with SCI, when type I diabetes mellitus coexists with SCI its management is more complicated.[4]

Diabetic Ketoacidosis [5-7]

|Diabetic ketoacidosis (DKA) is the most extreme manifestation of insulin deficiency. It occurs most commonly in type I diabetes but may also occur in type II diabetes. Many factors contribute to the development of DKA. Occasionally a patient has discontinued his insulin. Illness, such as infection or myocardial infarction, increases counterregulatory hormones, such as epinephrine and glucagon. These hormones result in resistance to insulin and may cause DKA.

|Type II diabetics, who have endogenous insulin secretion, are usually spared from ketoacidosis. Physiological stresses may increase insulin resistance permitting ketoacidosis to develop. Patients with SCI have a greater incidence of acute medical problems, such as infection and pulmonary embolism, which may predispose to DKA in type II diabetes. Patients with SCI often can't sense pain. Therefore, the only manifestation of a problem such as myocardial infarction may be ketoacidosis.

|Absolute or relative deficiency of insulin results in increased gluconeogenesis, muscle breakdown, lipolysis, and decreased glucose uptake into cells. Hyperglycemia results in an osmotic diuresis and dehydration. Much of the glucose that is produced by gluconeogenesis is excreted in the urine. The presence of renal failure, common in SCI, may worsen the degree of hyperglycemia. Decreased insulin results in mobilization of free fatty acids from fatty tissues. Decreased insulin and increased glucagon in turn increase the activity of the liver enzyme carnitine acyl transferase (CAT), which increases the flux of fatty acids in the mitochondria. In the mitochondria, fatty acids are metabolized to the ketone bodies acetoacetate, beta hydroxy butyrate, and acetone. Ketone bodies are weak acids. Bicarbonate is utilized in buffering them. If the anion is retained, then the anion gap ($Na + K - HCO_3 - CL$) increases (normal = 10 to 12 meq/l). The acidosis of DKA is most commonly that of an increased anion gap. However, if intravascular volume is normal and the glomerular filtration rate (GFR) is not decreased, the kidney may be able to excrete increased levels of ketone bodies as sodium and potassium salts and an increased anion gap may not be present. During treatment of DKA, bicarbonate is regenerated from ketone bodies. The loss of ketone bodies in the urine with retention of chloride may therefore result in persistence of hyperchloremic acidosis for several days after treatment is begun. The presence of renal failure in SCI, by impairing excretion of ketone bodies would make normal anion gap acidosis and persistent hyperchloremic acidosis less likely.

|Acidosis results in loss of potassium from cells. Osmotic diuresis results in depletion of total body potassium. Factors that are unique to patients with SCI may worsen body potassium depletion. Loss of sympathetic activity results in increased renin, angiotensin II, and aldosterone levels, which in turn leads to urinary potassium wasting. It therefore seems likely that these patients are prone to hypokalemia when DKA develops.

Clinical Manifestation of Diabetic Ketoacidosis in SCI
|Osmotic diuresis results in polydypsia and polyuria. About 30% of patients present with stupor or coma. Stupor and coma seem to be related to the serum osmolality level, which can be measured directly or calculated by the equation: (Serum osmolality = 2 Na (meq/l) + glucose (mg/dl)/18 + BUN (mg/dl)/2.8).

|Dehydration results in loss of skin turgor and hypotension. Abdominal pain and elevated serum amylase are common in DKA. However, with SCI, this symptom may not be present.

|Metabolic acidosis stimulates deep, regular ventilation (Kussmaul breathing). The ventilatory response to metabolic acidosis may be calculated from the equation: PCO_2 (mm mercury) = (serum bicarbonate meq/l) x 1.5 + 8. However the patients with SCI may not be able to increase their ventilation in response to acidosis. Therefore, in the patients with tetraplegia with impaired ventilatory reserve, the degree of acidosis in DKA may be more severe than in ambulatory patients.

Laboratory Findings
|The serum glucose is above 250 mg/dl in DKA. Arterial pH and low serum bicarbonate are low and serum and urine ketones are elevated. The serum phosphate may be low, normal, or high. The white blood count is commonly elevated even when infection is not present.

Treatment of Diabetic Ketoacidosis in SCI[9]
|The treatment of DKA consists in replacing insulin, fluid, and electrolyte losses. In addition, predisposing factors, such as infection, which is more common in patients with SCI, should be sought and treated. DKA should be treated in an intensive care unit with the patient on a cardiac monitor.

Insulin
|It has now been established that ketoacidosis does not cause insulin resistance. Therefore, high doses of insulin, which may cause hypoglycemia, are not required. Delivery of insulin at a rate of 4-10 units/hr. is sufficient to inhibit lipolysis and decrease blood glucose at a rate of 70 to 100 mg/dl/hr. Initially, a dose of .1 units/kg should be given intravenously. Insulin is then infused at a rate of 0.1 units/kg/hour. Glucose and electrolytes should determined at least hourly.

|If an intensive care unit is not available, the above doses of insulin may be given intramuscularly every hour. When the blood glucose is 250 to 300 mg/dl, D5W should be started to prevent further rapid fall in blood glucose. This is primarily to prevent hypoglycemia and cerebral edema. When ketonemia has cleared and the patient is eating, a routine dose of insulin can be established gradually with the use of a sliding scale (5 to 20 units of regular insulin SQ every 4 to 6 hours) to cover glucose levels above 200 mg/dl.

Fluid Replacement

|Intravascular volume is usually severely depleted in DKA. Hydration will improve insulin delivery to tissues and increase renal excretion of glucose, thereby lowering blood glucose. One liter of .45% or .9% saline is given in the first hour. It is uncertain which of these solutions is preferred. If the patient is hypotensive, .9% saline is preferred as the initial intravenous solution.

Potassium

|Patients with DKA are usually depleted of potassium; deficits of several hundred milliequivalents are not uncommon. Initiation of insulin and fluids, by increasing tissue uptake of potassium and increasing renal losses may further decrease serum potassium. Hypokalemia may cause arrhythmias and is one of the most common causes of death in DKA. Therefore, unless the serum potassium is elevated, potassium replacement should be begun at the beginning of treatment for DKA.

Bicarbonate

|Once insulin and fluid therapy is begun the body begins to regenerate lost bicarbonate. The use of bicarbonate in the treatment of DKA is controversial. Acidosis may affect cardiac function and impair insulin action. However, bicarbonate therapy, by increasing the pH decreases ventilatory drive, resulting in increased pCO_2, which diffuses into the brain and causes cerebrospinal fluid (CSF) acidosis.

|Because patients with tetraplegia have decreased ventilatory reserve, it is likely that CSF acidosis would be more severe in these patients. In addition, bicarbonate treatment may worsen hypokalemia. In moderately severe acidosis (pH 6.9 to 7.1) concomitant use of bicarbonate therapy has not been found to affect the outcome of DKA.[5] Bicarbonate should therefore not be used in this pH range. Because more severe acidosis presents added risk to the patient, bicarbonate should be given for pH below 6.9.

Phosphate

|Serum phosphate is often low in DKA. Low body phosphate results in low[2,3] diphosphoglycerate (DPG) levels, which impair oxygen delivery to tissues. In addition low phosphate may impair myocardial contractility. However, no controlled study has demonstrated a clinical benefit of phosphate on the treatment of DKA.[3] Furthermore phosphate may produce hypocalcemia.[3] Therefore, phosphate should not be administrated in DKA unless the serum phosphate is below 1 mg/dl.

Magnesium

|Serum magnesium is commonly low in DKA. If serum magnesium level is below 1 meq/l, intravenous magnesium should be given as 1 to 2 g of magnesium sulfate over 3 to 5 minutes followed by an infusion of 1 to 2 g/hour.

The treatment of DKA is summarized in Table I.

Table I **Treatment of Diabetic Ketoacidosis**

Fluids	Average fluid deficit is 5 to 7 liters. Give .9% or .45% saline 200 to 100 cc in the first hours depending on degree of dehydration. If hypovolemic shock is present initially, give .9% saline and plasma expanders. When the patient is out of shock and serum glucose is 250 to 300 mg/dl switch to D5W or D10W at a rate to maintain serum glucose 250 to 300 mg/dl.
Insulin	Regular Insulin. 0.1units/kg intravenous push, then 0.1units/kg IV per hour.
Potassium	Give none if serum potassium is above 4.5 meq/l. If potassium is below 4.5, give 20 to 40 meq KCl in first IV bottle. Monitor serum potassium at least every 3 to 4 hours. If potassium is below 4.5 and adequate urine output, give additional potassium as needed. *Avoid giving potassium through central lines.*
Bicarbonate	Give none if pH is greater than 6.9. If pH is below 6.9 give 100 meq sodium bicarbonate in first IV bottle. Determine serum HCO_3 every 2 hours. Repeat $NaHCO_3$ 100 meq if pH is below 7.
Phosphate	Give phosphate only if serum phosphate is below 1 mg/dl. Potassium replacement may be given as 1/2 potassium chloride and 1/2 potassium phosphate.

Problems in the Treatment of Ketoacidosis

|Hypoglycemia and hypokalemia are complications of therapy of DKA. These problems can be prevented with careful monitoring of the patient. Patients with DKA are susceptible to arterial and venous thrombosis; this risk is greater in patients with SCI especially in the acute phases of SCI. However, routine anticoagulation is not recommended.

|Infections are common in DKA and may be difficult to diagnose in patients with SCI.

|Cerebral edema is found most commonly in patients with DKA who have had a rapid fall in blood glucose during treatment. This condition is found most commonly in children with DKA. However, it may also occur in older patients and in patients with hyperosmolar hyperglycemic non-ketotic coma (HHNC). Typically the patient seems to be doing better during treatment, then convulses or becomes stuporous. This condition, which has a high mortality, is treated with intravenous mannitol to reduce CSF pressure. At autopsy cerebral edema is found. The mechanism of cerebral edema is uncertain. The theory of idiogenic brain osmoles suggests that during hyperglycemia an osmotically active substance accumulates in the brain increasing brain osmolality to prevent loss of brain water to hypertonic plasma.[10] However, with treatment of hyperglycemia plasma osmolality decreases. Brain osmolality takes longer to fall and therefore there is an osmotic gradient with a tendency for shift of fluid from the plasma to the brain. Because of this risk, too rapid fall in serum glucose below 250 to 300 mg/dl during treatment of DKA is to be avoided.

HHNC[5-7]

|In HHNC, hyperglycemia, dehydration and hyperosmolality occur. However, unlike DKA, in HHNC, acidosis is not present. HHNC is usually found in type II diabetes mellitus. In this disorder there is adequate insulin effect on the liver to prevent increased lipolysis and ketogenesis, but not enough to control blood glucose.

|Many medical conditions that occur in patients with SCI, including sepsis, congestive heart failure and cerebrovascular accidents, precipitate HHNC by increasing counterregulatory hormones. Drugs, such as phenytoin or glucocorticoids that decrease insulin secretion or promote insulin resistance may also precipitate HHNC.

Clinical Presentation

|Patients are often elderly. Like patients with DKA, they may present with polyuria and polydypsia and evidence of dehydration. Stupor and coma are commonly present. Probably in part because these patients are elderly and have coexistent medical problems this condition has a mortality of 40% to 70%.

|Serum glucose is markedly elevated. It is usually above 600 mg/dl and may be in the thousands. Serum osmolality is concomitantly very high. However, as opposed to DKA serum bicarbonate and potassium are usually normal. Increased serum osmolality results in shifts of water from tissues into the intravascular space producing "dilutional" hyponatremia.

Treatment

|The treatment of HHNC is similar to that of DKA. However, because acidosis is not present, use of bicarbonate is usually not a consideration. The goal of therapy is the replacement of volume loss, decreasing serum osmolality and treatment of concomitant medical problems.

|Insulin increases glucose uptake into cells and decreases gluconeogenesis. This is given at a rate of 0.05 to 0.1 units/kg IV/hr following an initial bolus of 0.05 to 0.1 units/kg IV. This will produce a gradual fall in serum glucose. When the serum glucose level reaches 250 to 300 mg/dl, D5W is begun at a rate of 80 to 100 cc/hour to prevent further fall in glucose.

|The initial fluid therapy is .45% saline or .9% saline. However, even .9% saline is hypotonic to the serum of patients with HHNC and will cause decline in serum osmolality. When the patient is hypotensive the initial bottle should be normal saline. Fluid replacement should be given cautiously with careful monitoring for congestive heart failure. In many situations, especially when underlying heart disease is present, a Swan-Ganz catheter for monitoring of right ventricular filling pressure is required.

|Because acidosis is not present and potassium depletion is usually less severe than in DKA, profound hypokalemia during treatment is less of a problem with HHNC than in DKA. However, if the serum potassium is normal or low, potassium should be added to each IV bottle.

Hypoglycemia

|Patients with SCI are especially predisposed to hypoglycemia. The most common causes of hypoglycemia are shown in Table II.

Table II **Causes of Hypoglycemia**[11]

I.	Use of insulin or oral hypoglycemic agents
II.	Liver disease
III.	Renal failure and dialysis
IV.	Starvation
V.	Reactive (postprandial) hypoglycemia
VI.	Adrenal insufficiency
VII.	Insulinoma
VIII.	Hypoglycemia secondary to large mesenchymal tumors

|Of these conditions, use of hypoglycemic drugs, and renal failure and dialysis occur with increased frequency in patients with SCI. With renal failure, metabolism of insulin by the kidney is impaired, which may promote hypoglycemia. Also, dialysis using dialysate that has low glucose concentration may produce transient hypoglycemia.

|The frequency of hypoglycemia from sulfonylureas or insulin is increased because of the increased incidence of type II diabetes mellitus. Hypoglycemia is unusual with sulfonylureas, however, it does occur. Hypoglycemia secondary to sulfonylureas occurs most commonly when the patient is starved, drinks alcohol (thereby inhibiting gluconeogenesis), or is using long-acting sulfonylureas, such as chlorpropamide. Chlorpropamide is totally excreted by the kidney. Impaired renal function may result in accumulation of chlorpropamide in the body and cause prolonged hypoglycemia. This drug should therefore be avoided in patients with SCI with renal impairment.

|Koivisto et al found that insulin absorption was increased in an exercising extremity when compared to absorption in a non-exercising extremity.[12] Alternating injection sites in patients with SCI from an exercising limb (e.g., arm) to a non-exercising limb (e.g., leg) may therefore produce wide swings in blood glucose and promote hypoglycemia. It is the policy of the SCI Unit at Hunter Holmes McGuire VAMC to inject insulin below the level of paralysis to avoid such wide swings in blood glucose.

|In addition to increased incidence of conditions causing hypoglycemia in patients with SCI, SCI may alter the presentation of hypoglycemia and impair recovery.

|Mathias et al compared the hormonal response to hypoglycemia in patients with tetraplegia with that in ambulatory patients.[13] Hypoglycemia produced an elevation of plasma epinephrine and norepinephrine in ambulatory patients, with concomitant symptoms of sweating, hunger, anxiety, and signs of tachycardia and hypertension. In contrast to ambulatory patients, hypoglycemia failed to produce a catecholamine response in patients with tetraplegia. Consequently sweating and anxiety were absent. Instead, patients with tetraplegia became confused and stuporous from decreased brain glucose (neuroglycopenia). Unlike in ambulatory patients whose blood pressure increased, insulin-induced hypoglycemia caused a profound fall in blood pressure in patients with tetraplegia. This is because of increased uptake of glucose and water into tissues. In spite of impaired sympathetic tone, patients with tetraplegia responded to hypoglycemia with tachycardia due to decreased vagal activity in response to falling blood pressure.

|Mathias also found that the normal suppression of endogenous insulin by hypoglycemia was blunted in patients with tetraplegia.[13] This is probably because of decreased sympathetic tone, which removes physiologic inhibition of insulin secretion. Failure of hypoglycemia to suppress insulin levels might predispose these patients to fasting hypoglycemia.

|Like Mathias, Palmer et al found that insulin hypoglycemia failed to provoke a catecholamine response in patients with tetraplegia.[14] However, the glucagon response and blood glucose responses were essentially normal. This would suggest that glucagon-stimulated glycogenolysis is critical in the recovery from hypoglycemia in patients with tetraplegia. In the ambulatory person, exercise results in release of catecholamines that help maintain serum glucose levels by stimulating gluconeogenesis and inhibiting muscle uptake of glucose. In patients with tetraplegia, lower body exercise may be facilitated by functional electrical stimulation. Such patients, who lack the sympathetic response to exercise, may be prone to hypoglycemia.

Treatment of Hypoglycemia
|Mild manifestations of hypoglycemia (sweating, hunger) can be treated with oral glucose. However, as mentioned above, these symptoms are often not present in patients with tetraplegia who instead become confused. Furthermore, motor dysfunction may impair the patient's ability to treat his hypoglycemia. Health care professionals must be alert to the development of hypoglycemia in patients with SCI, especially in those on insulin or sulfonylureas. Unexplained confusion in these patients should result in an immediate search for possible hypoglycemia.

|More severe hypoglycemia must be treated parenterally. Fifty cc of 50% glucose is given intravenously over 5 minutes. Any patient who reports to the emergency room in this manner, especially a patient with SCI, should be administrated IV glucose as treatment of possible hypoglycemia. In most cases this will reverse hypoglycemia and its symptoms. Blood glucose should continue to be monitored at ½- to 1-hour intervals. In situations where prolonged hypoglycemia is likely (e.g., use of chlorpropamide or in severe liver disease), an IV should be started for continuous delivery of 5% to 10% glucose at 80 to 120 cc/hour with determination of blood glucose at 1- to 2-hour intervals. In conditions such as end-stage liver disease or tumor hypoglycemia, intravenous glucose may be required indefinitely.

|Glucagon also will reverse hypoglycemia. Glucagon 1 mg is available in kits and is especially useful at home. The powdered glucagon can be rapidly reconstituted with diluent and injected subcutaneously, intramuscularly or intravenously. However, in situations where liver glycogen stores are depleted (such as in starvation or cirrhosis) glucagon may be ineffective in raising the blood glucose. Furthermore, certain drugs, such as indomethacin may impair glycogenolysis.[15]

|Once hypoglycemia is resolved its cause should be sought. Often the cause is obvious (e.g., a missed meal in an insulin-treated diabetic). In this instance, greater attention to caloric intake or reduced insulin dose may be all that is required to prevent further episodes. Situations in which the etiology of hypoglycemia is unclear require further testing.

|Unless hypoglycemia is due to endogenous insulin (i.e., insulinoma) or exogenous insulin, serum insulin levels are suppressed. The finding of fasting hypoglycemia with an inappropriately elevated serum insulin level suggests one of those causes.

Conclusion

|Hyperglycemic and hypoglycemic emergencies occur with increased frequency in patients with SCI and their course may be altered by impairment in the sympathetic nervous system. Patients with DKA present with hyperglycemia, low serum pH and bicarbonate, and ketonemia. DKA is treated with insulin and cautious fluid and electrolyte replacement.

|In HHNC, acidosis is not present. HHNC is treated with insulin and hypotonic fluids. In both DKA and HHNC, underlying medical conditions, such as infection, should be sought.

|Hypoglycemia is most commonly due to the use of hypoglycemic drugs in diabetic patients. In SCI the usual adrenergic signs and symptoms may not be present. Hypoglycemia is treated with oral and parenteral glucose and parenteral glucagon.

References

1. Schmitt JK, Adler RA. Endocrine-metabolic consequences if spinal cord injury. *Phys Med. Rehab, State Art Reviews* 1987;1:425-441.

2. Duckworth WC, Solomon SS, Jallipalli P, et al. Glucose intolerance due to insulin resistance in patients with spinal cord injuries. *Diabetes* 1980;29:906-910.

3. Bauman W, Spungen A. Disorders of carbohydrates and lipid metabolism in veterans with paraplegia or quadriplegia: a model of premature aging. *Metabolism* 1994;43:749-756.

4. Barlascini CU, Schmitt JK, Adler RA. Insulin pump treatment of type I diabetics in a patient with C6 quadriplegia. *Arch Phys Med Rehab* 1989;7:58-60.

5. Silverberg JD, Kreisberg RA. Hyperglycemic disorders. *Problems in Critical Care* 1990;4:355-371.

6. Kitabchi AE, Murphy MB. Diabetic ketoacidosis and hyperosmolar hyperglycemic nonketotic coma. *Med Clin NA* 1988;72:1545-1563.

7. Unger R, Foster D. Diabetes Mellitus. In: Wilson J, Foster D, Krouenberg H, Larsen P, (Eds) *Williams Textbook of Endocrinology*, WB Saunders: Philadelphia, 1998:pp. 973-1207.

8. Oh MS, Banerji MA, Carroll HJ. The mechanism of hyperchloremic acidosis during the recovery phase of diabetic ketoacidosis. *Diabetes* 1980;30:310-313.

9. Kitabchi AE, Fisher JN. Insulin therapy of diabetic ketoacidosis: physiologic versus pharmacologic doses of insulin and their roles of administration. In: Brownlee M. (Ed). *Handbook of Diabetes Mellitus*, Garland ATPM Press: New York, 1981:pp. 95-140.

10. Arieff Al, Kleeman CR. Studies on the mechanism of cerebral edema in diabetic comas. *J Clin Invest* 1973;52:571-583.

11. Comi RJ, Gordon P. Hypoglycemic disorders in the adult. In: Becker K (Ed). *Principles and Practice of Endocrinology and Metabolism*. JP Lippincott: Philadelphia, 1990:pp. 1198-1211.

12. Koivisto V, Felig P. Effects of leg exercise on insulin absorption in diabetic patients. *N Eng J Med* 1978;298:79-83.

13. Mathias CJ, Frankel HL, Turner RC, et al. Physiological responses to hypoglycemia in spinal man. *Paraplegia* 1980;17:319-326.

14. Palmer JP, Henry DP, Benson JW, et al. Glucagon response to hypoglycemia in sympathectomized man. *J Clin Invest* 1976;57:522-525.

15. Barlascini CO, Schmitt JK. Indomethacin, hypoglycemia, quadriplegia. *Arch Phys Med Rehab* 1987;68:746.

FLUID AND ELECTROLYTE DISORDERS

and Acute Renal Failure in Patients With SCI

James K. Schmitt, MD; Meena Midha, MD; Norma D. McKenzie, MD

CHAPTER NINE ■■■■■■■■■■■■■■■■

|Patients with spinal cord injury (SCI) are predisposed to disorders of fluid and electrolyte balance. Major causes of abnormalities in fluid and electrolyte homeostasis are acute and chronic renal failure, which occur with increased frequency in these patients. However, in addition to renal problems, patients with SCI may develop a variety of problems, such as infections, which alter the body's handling of fluids and electrolytes. Furthermore, the clinical presentation of disorders, such as hyponatremia, may be altered in patients with SCI making the diagnosis of these problems more difficult.

Normal Fluid and Electrolyte Homeostasis[1]

|In ambulatory persons, body water comprises about 60% of body weight. Two-thirds of body water is intracellular and the remainder is extracellular. Over 95% of sodium is extracellular. Sodium is accompanied by its associated anions, principally chloride and bicarbonate. Body water and electrolytes are maintained by humoral elements and the kidneys. Sodium and water balance are closely related. The serum osmolality is maintained within a narrow range. The serum osmolality may be calculated from the equation: osmolality = (2 Na + glucose/18+ BUN/2.8), where the serum sodium concentration is expressed in meq/l and the blood urea nitrogen (BUN) and glucose concentrations are expressed as mg/dl.

|Increases in osmolality are sensed by osmoreceptors within the hypothalamus. As little as a 2% increase in osmolality stimulates antidiuretic hormone (ADH) release from the posterior pituitary and thirst increases. Endothelin 1 released by the posterior pituitary modulates ADH levels. ADH results in increased free water absorption by the distal tubules, which will lower the serum osmolality toward normal. Conversely decreased serum osmolality results in decreased secretion of ADH, leading to increased excretion of free water and an increase in the serum osmolality. Hypovolemia, which is sensed by baroreceptors, also increases ADH secretion. When extracellular fluid (ECF) is reduced by more than 10%, non-osmotic ADH release occurs. In addition, hypovolemia activates the renin-angiotensin-aldosterone axis. Angiotensin II raises blood pressure by vasoconstriction, stimulates thirst, and increases serum aldosterone levels. Aldosterone increases sodium reabsorption and potassium excretion by the kidney.

|In ambulatory persons, increased activity of the sympathetic nervous system, by increasing blood pressure and cardiac output protects the body from the effects of hypovolemia. However, in patients with tetraplegia this response to hypovolemia and shock may be impaired. The above mechanisms for maintenance of intravascular volumes are therefore more important in patients with tetraplegia.

|When intravascular volume becomes too high, prostaglandin E2 (PGE2) and atrial natriuretic peptide increase. PGE2 is a direct antagonist of the tubular effects of ADH, inhibits tubular sodium absorption and is a renal vasodilator. Atrial natriuretic peptide, which is released from the atria, also has been identified in the central nervous system (CNS). Atrial natriuretic peptide suppresses ADH release, inhibits aldosterone secretion and increases renal blood flow. It also may block collecting duct and renal water absorption directly. The net result of these actions is to increase renal losses of water and sodium.

Effect of SCI on Fluid and Electrolyte Balance [2-4]

|ECF volume is relatively increased and intracellular volume decreased in patients with tetraplegia.[5] These patients experience a nocturnal naturesis, which may in part be due to increased atrial natriuretic peptide in the supine position.[6]

|Hyponatremia occurs frequently in patients with SCI. The incidence of hyponatremia is 10% to 15% as compared to 1% to 2% of the general population. The reason for this increase is uncertain. Lack of sympathetic tone results in pooling of blood in the capacitance vessels. Loss of sympathetic activity combined with venous pooling results in orthostatic hypotension. This loss of effective blood volume results in increased activity of the renin-angiotensin system and release of ADH. ADH is also released during periods of stress, such as infections, which occur frequently in patients with SCI.

|As was previously stated, PGE2, which is secreted by the medullary interstitial cells, antagonizes the effect of ADH. It has been speculated that in patients with SCI who have interstitial damage, reduced PGE2 may result in augmented ADH effect. However, Sica et al found no correlation between PGE2 excretion, renal function, urine volume, or sodium concentration.[5] In addition to the above factors, many other conditions including alcoholism, sepsis, liver disease, pneumonia, malnutrition, and hemorrhagic pancreatitis result in increased ADH levels.

Diagnosis of Hyponatremia[1,2,4]

|Hyponatremia may be due to a true decrease in serum sodium concentration. Hyponatremia may also occur with a normal serum osmolality. This "pseudohyponatremia" may occur with hypertriglyceridema and proteinemia. These disorders increase the non-sodium-containing fraction of plasma causing pseudohyponatremia. Before initiating treatment for hyponatremia the provider should be certain that the plasma is not lipemic. Osmotically active substances, such as glucose, when elevated, may cause shifts of fluids into the intravascular space causing hyponatremia.

|A true reduction in serum sodium often has clinical significance. Manifestations of hyponatremia generally don't occur until the plasma sodium falls below 120 meq/l. Clinical findings of hyponatremia include lethargy, malaise, and muscle cramps. With lack of treatment or increasing severity of hyponatremia, seizures, coma, psychosis, and permanent neurological damage and death may occur.

|True hyponatremia has three forms: that with increased ECF volume; that with normal body water; and that with decreased ECF volume.

|Most cases of hyponatremia are due to dilution (excess body water). Hyponatremia with volume excess and edema may result from renal failure, congestive heart failure, nephrotic syndrome, or cirrhosis. Impaired free water excretion results in volume overload and reduction of the serum sodium. Treatment of this form of hyponatremia is treatment of the underlying disorder and restriction of daily fluid intake to 500 to 1000 cc/day. Loop diuretics, such as furosemide, increase free water excretion.

|Hyponatremia with normal ECF or slightly increased volume is usually due to inappropriate ADH release. Hyponatremia with reduced plasma osmolality is present. In spite of the hyponatremia, the urine is inappropriately concentrated (greater than 200 milliosmoles/kg). Urinary sodium is elevated. Syndrome of inappropriate antidiuretic hormone (SIADH) may be due to certain tumors, especially of the lung, pulmonary, and CNS diseases and some drugs (e.g., amitryptiline).

|Patients with SCI often drink large amounts of water to prevent kidney stones. This results in hyponatremia. However, this condition can be distinguished from SIADH by the low osmolality of the urine as compared to the high osmolality in SIADH. In volume expansion urinary excretion of uric acid increases, resulting in hypouricemia. Conversely, when volume is contracted renal urate excretion decreases and serum urate increases. Chronic hyponatremia secondary to SIADH should be treated with fluid restriction of 500 to 1000 cc/day. Acute or symptomatic hyponatremia with a serum sodium rate of less than 110 to 115 meq/l should be treated more aggressively. Furosemide 1mg/kg given intravenously increases free water excretion. Replacement of electrolyte losses can be made with .9% saline. Rarely 3% saline is required. If it is given, 3% saline should be administered at 25 to 100 ml/hour with careful observation for fluid overload and too rapid a rise in serum sodium concentration. During the acute treatment of hyponatremia, serum sodium rise should not exceed 20 meq/l during the first 48 hours of therapy.

|Hyponatremia may also be associated with decreased ECF. This may occur in situations where total body sodium is depleted in excess of water loss as in conditions such as vomiting and diarrhea. The major manifestations are usually those of volume depletion rather than hyponatremia. The treatment is expansion of volume with isotonic saline and correction of the underlying condition (e.g., diarrhea).

|Rapid treatment of hyponatremia should be avoided. Rapid correction of hyponatremia has been reported to cause central pontine myelinolysis, and extrapontine myelinolysis, which may result in altered mental status, decreased speech, oral-buccal-lingual movements, pseudobulbar palsy, nystagmus, cranial nerve palsies, and flaccid tetraplegia.[7] Central pontine myelinolysis and extrapontine myelinolysis may be more difficult to diagnose in the patients with SCI than in the ambulatory subject. These disorders are felt to be due to fluid shifts in the brainstem due to rapidly changing sodium levels.

Hypernatremia[1]

|Hypernatremia is usually due to loss of hypotonic fluid from the body by mechanisms such as sweating and insensible losses. Patients with SCI who may lack appropriate thermoregulation and may be unable to drink without assistance, are predisposed to this form of hypernatremia. Less common causes of hypernatremia are central or nephrogenic diabetes insipidus. Rarely, transient hypernatremia is due to ingestion of hypertonic saline.

|Manifestations of hypernatremia include tremulousness, irritability, ataxia, spasticity, mental confusion, seizures, and coma. As with hyponatremia, acute hypernatremia is more likely to be symptomatic than chronic hypernatremia. Physical findings may be those of dehydration including dry mucous membranes, poor skin turgor and a postural fall in blood pressure. This last physical finding may be difficult to interpret in patients with tetraplegia. Patients with a serum sodium greater than 160 meq/l for more than 48 hours have a 60% mortality rate.

|The treatment of hypernatremia is replacement of water. Total body water (TBW) may be calculated from the equation:

$$\text{TBW (liters)} = 0.6 \times \text{current body weight (kg)}$$

$$\text{The desired TBW} = \frac{\text{Measured serum Na (meq/l)}}{\text{Normal serum Na (meq/l)}} \times \text{current TBW}$$

$$\text{The body water deficit} = \text{desired TBW} - \text{current TBW}$$

|One half of the calculated water deficit should be administered in the first 24 hours. The remaining deficit should be corrected in the next 1 to 2 days. The serum sodium concentration should not be corrected at a rate greater than 1 meq/hour. Rapid correction of hypernatremia is dangerous and may cause lethargy and seizures secondary to cerebral edema.

|Patients with SCI have been reported to have increased total body water due to decreased muscle mass. However, at this time, it seems unnecessary to correct the above equation for changes in body water in patients with SCI.

Potassium Homeostasis[1]

|Potassium is largely intracellular. Therefore a 1-meq/l fall in serum potassium indicates a 300-meq decrease in total body potassium. The major organ for the regulation of serum potassium is the kidney. Approximately 90% of dietary potassium is excreted into the distal convoluted tubule and collecting duct. The major factor modulating renal potassium excretion is aldosterone. Other factors promoting renal potassium wasting are increased delivery of sodium to the collecting duct, increased fluid flow to the distal convoluted tubule, alkalosis and increased excretion of non-reabsorbable solutes. Because renal adaptation to excess potassium intake occurs in a short period of time (24 to 36 hours), hyperkalemia from increased potassium intake is unusual in individuals with normal renal function. However, the renal adaptation to reduced potassium intake takes longer to occur (7 to 10 days).

|Lean muscle mass is reduced in patients with SCI. Ninety-eight percent of total body potassium is located in lean tissue. Therefore, total body potassium is reduced in these patients.[8] Because the renin-angiotensin II-aldosterone axis is increased in patients with tetraplegia, these patients may be predisposed to hypokalemia, especially when they are placed on diuretics.[9,10]

|The use of antibiotics, such as carbenicillin and gentamycin, promotes renal wasting of potassium. Patients with SCI also may experience gastrointestinal (GI) potassium losses from vomiting and other causes, such as laxative use. Initiation of insulin therapy in the patients with SCI who also have diabetes may cause hypokalemia by shifts of potassium into the intracellular space as may metabolic and respiratory alkalosis.

Signs and Symptoms of Hypokalemia

|The most worrisome manifestations of potassium depletion are cardiac. Electrocardiogram (ECG) manifestations of hypokalemia include sagging of the ST segment, depression of the T Wave and elevation of the U Wave. Hypokalemia may also cause cardiac ectopy including premature ventricular and atrial contractions. Hypokalemia in patients treated with digitalis may precipitate lethal arrhythmias including ventricular tachycardia and fibrillation. With serum potassium levels of 2 to 2.5 meq/l muscular weakness occurs. With lower serum potassium levels, paralysis and respiratory insufficiency and death may occur. This effect is especially significant in the patient with tetraplegia who already has significant respiratory compromise. Loss of large amounts of potassium from muscle (e.g., excess sweating) may result in rhabdomyolysis, myoglobinuria, and acute renal failure. Potassium depletion may also produce paralytic ileus, a condition to which patients with SCI are predisposed. Hypokalemia may also produce renal tubular damage, which can result in nephrogenic diabetes insipidus and dehydration.

Treatment of Hypokalemia [1]

|In most cases oral replacement is adequate. Remember that in a patient with normal acid base balance, a decrease in serum potassium of 1 meq/l indicates a total body deficit of 300 meq. Unless the patient is on digitalis or there are cardiac manifestations, serum potassium levels greater than 3 meq/l may be treated with oral supplements. Forty to 100 meq of potassium citrate or gluconate may be administered in divided doses (oral potassium chloride solutions are not well tolerated because of gastrointestinal irritation). Enteric-coated potassium chloride tablets should be avoided because of the possibility of small bowel perforation, which may be especially problematic in the patients with SCI. In more severe hypokalemia or if the patient cannot take oral medications, intravenous therapy must be given. Potassium should never be administered through a central line as it may cause asystole. If the serum potassium level is greater than 2.5 meq/l and there are no ECG changes, potassium should not be administered at a rate greater than 10 meq/hour or in a concentration greater than 30 meq/l.

|The maximum daily amount of potassium given, usually should not exceed 100 to 200 meq. If the serum potassium is less than 2 meq/l, or ECG or other chemical manifestations occur, more emergent treatment is necessary. Intravenous potassium may be administered at a rate up to 40 meq/hour in concentrations up to 60 meq/l. In such situations, treatment in an ICU with continuous ECG monitoring is imperative. Serum potassium should be determined every 4 hours. In hypokalemic emergencies, potassium should be administered in glucose-free solutions, as administration of glucose will decrease serum potassium further.

|Once potassium is repleted, the patient should be placed on daily replacement dose commensurate with his loss. For example, a patient on diuretics usually requires 20 to 60 meq replacement per day.

|In the treatment of hypokalemia, the patient's acid base status must be considered. Because acidosis shifts potassium out of cells, hypokalemia in association with metabolic acidosis, such diabetic ketoacidosis, indicates profound total body potassium depletion. With the treatment of the cause of acidosis (e.g., insulin in diabetic ketoacidosis) serum potassium will decrease further. In such patients the cardiac rhythm and serum potassium should be monitored extremely closely. Hypokalemia may cause death in diabetic ketoacidosis (DKA). Conversely, hypokalemia with normal body potassium may be secondary to alkalosis. In this situation, treating the cause of the alkalosis may be all that is required to relieve the hypokalemia.

Hyperkalemia [1]

|Hyperkalemia is usually due to decreased renal excretion or shifts of potassium out of cells as in conditions such as DKA.

|The most common causes of decreased renal excretion are acute and chronic renal failure. Other causes are: decreased aldosterone production, such as occurs in Addison's disease; potassium-sparing diuretics; use of non-steroidal anti-inflammatory drugs (NSAIDS) and angiotensin-converting enzyme inhibitors (especially in patients with renal disease); another cause is hyporeninemic hypoaldosteronism. Transcellular shifts of potassium may occur in acidosis, cellular destruction, such as rhabdomyolysis, and with induction of depolarizing muscle paralysis with drugs, such as succinylcholine. Because the kidneys rapidly adapt to increased potassium intake, increased intake alone is rarely a cause of hyperkalemia. Pseudo-hyperkalemia may occur in situations when clotting of blood occurs at the time it is drawn, as potassium is released from cells. In this circumstance, although the serum potassium is elevated, the plasma level is normal.

|The most dangerous consequences of hyperkalemia relate to the cardiovascular system. Peaking of the T Wave, the earliest manifestation of hyperkalemia occurs when the serum potassium exceeds 6.5 meq/l. With higher levels of serum potassium (7 to 8 meq/l) prolongation of the PR interval, loss of P Waves and widening of the QRS complex occurs. At still higher levels of serum potassium (greater than 8 to 10 meq/l) a sine wave pattern on ECG may occur, followed by asystole.

|The treatment of elevated serum potassium depends on the severity of hyperkalemia. With serum potassium levels above 6 to 6.5 meq/l, the mainstay of treatment is to shift potassium out of the extravascular space into the intracellular space. Administration of 25 g of glucose intravenously with 10 units of regular insulin over 30 minutes rapidly reduces serum potassium. Administration of glucose without insulin may transiently worsen hyperkalemia.

|Sodium bicarbonate also shifts potassium into the cells, especially in acidosis. One ampule of 7.5% Na HCO$_3$ (44.6 meq Na HCO$_3$) may be given intravenously over 5 minutes and repeated if ECG changes persist. Sodium bicarbonate should be administered cautiously, especially in patients with renal insufficiency as circulatory overload and hypernatremia may occur. Potassium may also be shifted to the intracellular compartment using beta 2 agonists, such as albuterol.

|In situations of severe cardiotoxicity (e.g., P Waves are absent and QRS complexes are widened), calcium gluconate 10 to 20 ml of 10% solution should be administered over 10 to 20 minutes intravenously. Calcium does not lower serum potassium but counteracts the cardiac effects. In such a situation the patient should be on constant ECG monitoring.

|Once potassium has been shifted intracellularly, measures to remove it from the body should be instituted. Kayexalate is a cation-exchange resin that binds about 1 meq of potassium for each gram of resin. Twenty grams of kayexalate may be given in a 20% solution of sorbitol 4 times daily. The sorbitol induces diarrhea, which aids in the resin passage through the GI tract. Kayexalate also may be given by enema with 100 g of resin suspended in 200 ml of 20% sorbitol. Kayexalate and sorbitol may be all that is required in the treatment of mild hyperkalemia (less than 6 meq/l). Diuretics, such as furosemide (40 mg IV), will also lower body potassium levels.

|In some disorders, such as severe burns or massive trauma in which tissue damage results in such high release of potassium that resins cannot remove it adequately, hemodialysis or peritoneal dialysis may be indicated, especially in patients with coexistent renal impairment.

Hypomagnesemia[11]

|Hypomagnesemia is found in 9% to 11% of hospital patients. Etiologies include poor oral intake, alcoholism, loss from draining wounds, and decubiti. Several drugs cause renal magnesium wasting (diuretics, aminoglyosides, and cisplatinum). Hypomagnesemia may result in hypocalcemia and hypokalemia that are refractory to therapy, anorexia, vomiting, mental confusion, tremor, seizures, ECG changes, and arrhythmias. Severe hypomagnesemia (i.e., symptomatic hypomagnesemia, or a serum magnesium level below 1 meq/l) may be treated with 1 to 2 grams of $Mg\,SO_4$ (2 to 4 ml of 50% solution) by continuous IV infusion.

Acute Renal Failure[4, 12, 13]

|Chronic renal failure is one of the most frequent causes of death in patients with SCI.[4] The most common etiologies are chronic pyelonephritis, amyloidosis, calculous disease, and obstructive uropathy.

|Acute renal failure also occurs more frequently in patients with SCI than in ambulatory subjects. Often acute renal failure is superimposed upon chronic renal failure, which adds to the difficulty of the diagnosis. Acute renal failure may be prerenal, intrarenal, or postrenal.

|Prerenal failure may be due to decreased intravascular volume, ineffective arterial volume (pressure) or renal artery occlusion.

|Postrenal failure is due to occlusion of the ureters, the uretha or renal vein occlusion.

|Intrarenal failure may be due to a variety of causes including vasculitis, glomerulonephritis, tubular necrosis secondary to hypotension, sepsis, deposition of hemoglobin, myoglobin, uric acid, calcium and other substances, and numerous nephrotoxins.

|Renal failure may be oliguric (urine output less than 30 ml/hour) or nonoliguric. The history and physical given clues to the cause of acute renal failure. Decreased urine output in a patient with massive GI bleeding should make the provider suspicious of prerenal failure. Oliguria in a diabetic who has undergone a radiographic procedure using contrast should raise the suspicion of renal failure secondary to contrast agents. Anuria in a patient with tetraplegia with an indwelling catheter should raise the suspicion of an occluded catheter.

|The urinalysis is often useful. Hyaline casts suggest prerenal disease. In postrenal disease white blood cells may be present if infection is present. In intrarenal failure, red blood cell casts suggest glomerular disease. Tubular cells suggest tubular disease.

|In prerenal azotemia, the kidneys avidly retain water and sodium. The urine osmolality is therefore high (greater than 500 milliosmoles/kg H_2O), urinary sodium low (less than 20 meq/l). The urine/plasma creatinine ratio is greater than 20 and the plasma BUN/creatinine ratio is increased. The fractional excretion of sodium is useful, defined as:

$$\frac{\text{Urine (Na)/serum (Na)}}{\text{Urine creatinine/serum creatinine}} \times 100$$

|A fractional excretion of sodium less than 1% suggests a prerenal cause of renal failure. A fractional excretion of greater than 1% suggests acute tubular injury.

|When postrenal failure is suspected, a Foley catheter may relieve obstruction. However, if possible, indwelling catheters should be avoided, as they may cause infection. If clinical evidence suggests prerenal failure, a fluid challenge of 500 cc to 1000 cc of saline should be administered. In patients with congestive heart failure, a Swan-Ganz catheter may need to be placed to monitor filling pressure.

|Ultrasonography is useful in diagnosing postrenal obstruction, which may cause hydronephrosis and bladder enlargement. Enlarged kidneys on ultrasound examination indicate intrinsic renal damage. Small kidneys indicate underlying chronic disease. A combination of fluid challenge (500 ml of saline) and 40 to 80 mg of furosemide may reverse renal failure or convert oliguric renal failure to nonoliguric renal failure. Saline challenges should not be administered to patients with edema or ascites.

Features of Acute Renal Failure

|Sodium and water retention results in weight gain and edema. The serum creatinine rises at a rate of 1.0 to 2.0 mg/dl/day in ambulatory patients with acute renal failure. With increased muscle breakdown and myoglobinuria, the serum creatinine rises more rapidly. Because patients with SCI have decreased muscle mass, their creatinine rise will tend to be lower than in ambulatory patients. In intrinsic renal disease, the BUN creatinine ratio is maintained at 10:1. With prerenal conditions the ratio is usually 20:1 or greater. Hyperkalemia, metabolic acidosis, hyperuricemia, and hyperphosphatemia from impaired renal excretion occur.

|Increasing serum phosphate binds calcium and causes hypocalcemia. After several days anemia from impaired erythropoietin production develops. Unexcreted waste products result in the uremic syndrome, which is manifested by anorexia, nausea, vomiting, nervous irritability, hyperreflexia, seizures, and coma.

Treatment of Acute Renal Failure

|Reversible causes should be corrected. Relief of lower urinary tract obstruction usually results in dramatic improvement in renal function.

|Nephrotoxic drugs, such as gentamycin and NSAIDS, should be discontinued. In pre-renal failure, restoration of blood volume and sometimes uses of pressors such as dopamine will improve renal function. In a patient with myocardial disease, the placement of a pulmonary artery line for monitoring filling pressures and cardiac output may be necessary.

|Daily weights should be measured. A general guideline for fluid replacement is to give the patient 500 ml of fluid plus the amount of urine excreted in the past 24 hours. Dietary protein should be limited to 0.8 g/kg/day. Energy from carbohydrate and fats should supply 35 kcal/day. Remember that the ideal body weight of a patient with tetraplegia is .6 times that of an ambulatory patient and the ideal body weight of a patient with paraplegia is .8 times that of an ambulatory patient. Energy requirements should therefore be adjusted accordingly.

|Blood pressure should be determined every 4 to 6 hours and electrolytes should be measured at least daily. Hyperphosphatemia should be corrected by use of phosphate binders and hyperkalemia is corrected as previously described.

|Hemodialysis or peritoneal dialysis are required for refractory acidosis, hyperkalemia, pulmonary edema, azotemia with BUN greater than 100 mg/dl, encephalopathy, seizures, bleeding, pericarditis, or uremic enteropathy.

|In postrenal and prerenal acute renal failure, recovery is common if perfusion is restored or obstruction is relieved. Intrinsic causes of renal failure have a more variable prognosis. Some cases of glomerulonephritis and vasculitis may respond to steroids and other immunosuppressive agents. In other cases recovery may not occur and chronic renal failure ensues. This may be especially likely in patients with SCI who have underlying chronic renal failure prior to the acute insult.

Prevention of Acute Renal Failure

|Patients with SCI are at high risk for acute renal failure and providers should be vigilant to prevent this sometimes fatal complication. Avoidance of indwelling catheters prevents infection and reduces risk of renal stones. Extra care should be taken in the use of nephrotoxic drugs, especially in patients who have underlying chronic renal disease. Ensurance of adequate hydration during procedures using contrast agents will prevent renal failure.

Conclusion

|Disorders of the kidney and electrolytes occur with increased frequency in patients with SCI. Prerenal failure secondary to disorders, such as dehydration, intrinsic renal failure from radiographic contrast agents and postrenal failure, all are increased in patients with SCI. Prerenal failure is corrected by administration of fluids. Postrenal failure may be reversed by relief of obstruction.

|Hyponatremia is most commonly due to conditions in which free water excretion is impaired, such as liver disease and SIADH. Most cases of hyponatremia may be treated by water restriction. Severe cases may require administration of saline and furosemide. Rapid correction of hyponatremia may produce central and extrapontine myelinolysis.

|Hypernatremia is usually due to dehydration and is treated with administration of fluids.

|Hypokalemia is usually due to excess renal excretion of potassium and is treated by potassium replacement.

|Hyperkalemia is due to renal failure, drugs that inhibit potassium excretion, and conditions that displace potassium from cells, such as acidosis. Hyperkalemia is treated by blocking the acute effects of potassium on the myocardium with calcium; shifting potassium into cells with bicarbonate, insulin and glucose; and removing potassium from the body (kayexalate).

References

1. Kokko JP. Disorders of fluid, volume electrolyte and acid base balance. *Cecil's Textbook of Medicine*. Bennett J, Plum F (Eds). WB Saunders: Philadelphia, 1996, pp. 522-525.

2. Sica D, Midha M, Zawada E, et al. Hyponatremia in Spinal Cord Injury. *J Am Paraplegia Soc* 1990;13:78-83.

3. Sica D, Midha M. Zawada E, et al. Prostaglandin E_2 excretion in spinal cord injury patients. *J Am Paraplegia Soc* 1984;7:27-29.

4. Stacy W, Midha M. The kidney in the spinal cord injury patient. *Phys Med Rehabil* 1987;1:415-423.

5. Cardus D, McTaggert WG. Total body water and its distribution in men with spinal cord injury. *Arch Phys Med Rehabil* 1984;65:509-512.

6. Sica D, Midha M, Aronoff G, et al. Atrial natriuretic factor in spinal cord injury. *Arch Phys Med Rehabil* 1993;74:969-972.

7. Moore K, Midha M. Extrapontine myelinolysis in a tetraplegic patient. Case Report. *Spinal Cord* 1997;35:332-334.

8. Spungen AM, Bauman W, Wang J, et al. The relationship between total body potassium and resting energy expenditure in individuals with paraplegia. *Arch Phys Med Rehabil* 1993;74:965-968.

9. Mathias CJ, Christensen N, Corbett J, et al. Plasma catecholamines, plasma renin activity and plasma aldoseterone in tetraplegic man, horizontal and tilted. *Clin Sci Med* 1975;49:291-299.

10. Schmitt JK, Koch KS, Midha M. Profound hypotension in a tetraplegic patient following angiotensin-converting enzyme inhibitor lisinopril. *Paraplegia* 1994;32: 871-874.

11. Berkelhammer C, Bear RA. A clinical approach to common electrolyte problems IV hypomagnesemia. *Can Med Assoc J* 1985;132:360-368.

12. Mitch WE. Acute renal failure. In: *Cecil's Textbook of Medicine*. Bennett JC, Plum F (Eds). WB Saunders: Philadelphia, 1996, pp. 552-556.

13. Schmitt J, Midha M, McKenzie ND. Medical Complications of Spinal Cord Disease. In: Young R, Woolsey R (Eds). *Diagnosis and Management of Disorders of the Spinal Cord*. WB Saunders: Philadelphia, 1995, pp. 297-316.

James K. Schmitt, MD;
Brent A. Armstrong, MD

|PULMONARY EMBOLISM

and Deep Venous Thrombosis in Patients With SCI

CHAPTER TEN ▰▰▰▰▰▰▰▰▰▰▰▰▰▰

|Virchows's triad of risk factors for deep venous thrombosis (DVT) is hypercoagulability, decreased blood flow, and injury to the vessel. At least the first two of these factors are present in patients with spinal cord injury (SCI). Abnormalities in coagulation factors that increase the risk of thrombosis have been found in spinal cord disease. Myllynen et al found that factor VIII antigen (which reflects endothelial damage) and factor VIII procoagulant activity increase during the 10 to 12 days of immobilization in acute SCI.[1] These researchers also found that a ratio of factor VII antigen to procoagulant activity of greater than 2:1 accurately predicted the development of DVT. Petaja and colleagues found fibrinolytic activity to be decreased during the first 24 hours after spinal trauma.[2] Vaziri et al found that antithrombin III levels were lower in patients with SCI who had end-stage renal disease than in ambulatory patients with end-stage renal disease.[3] Factor VII and VIII activities were also found to be higher in patients with SCI who had renal failure when compared to controls. In addition to these factors, tissue damage at the time of SCI increases platelet number and adherence to surfaces.

|Radiolabeled fibrinogen and venography are sensitive ways of diagnosing DVT. Using these methods Myllynen et al found that 64% of patients with SCI had DVT.[4] In comparison, none of a group of non-paralyzed patients had DVT. This data demonstrates the importance of immobilization as a cause of DVT. After several weeks the risk of DVT decreases. This is because the effects of the acute injury on the coagulation cascade diminish, and spasticity, which increases venous return, begins to develop.

Diagnosis of DVT

|The classic finding of calf pain, which is common in ambulatory patients, is usually not present in patients with SCI who lack sensation in this area.[5] Leg swelling may be interpreted as being due to some other cause, such as congestive heart failure or nephrosis. When an unexplained fever occurs in a patient with SCI, the diagnosis of DVT should be considered.[6] Unilateral venous stasis edema may mimic a venous thrombosis, as may cellulitis, heterotopic ossification, and popliteal cysts. Spontaneous hematomas may also mimic DVT, especially in patients on antiplatelet agents, such as aspirin, or on heparin or warfarin. When the femoral and iliac veins are involved by DVT there may be tenderness over these veins in ambulatory patients.[5] However, these findings are usually not present in patients with SCI.

|Duplex doppler ultrasonography is a sensitive non-invasive test for the diagnosis of DVT.[7] Each venous segment is evaluated for incompressibility of the vein during probe pressure. An acute clot usually cannot be visualized directly. However, abnormal Doppler flow signals, including absence of blood flow, loss of flow variation with respiration, and failure to increase flow velocity with distal augmentation provide reliable evidence of the presence or absence of a clot. Impedance plethysmography is based on the principle that thrombosis results in decreased venous flow, which decreases an electrical signal. Impedance plethysmography detects proximal venous obstruction with a sensitivity as high as 98% but is unreliable in the detection of calf thrombi. Venous Doppler ultrasound detects thrombi in the common femoral or popliteal veins in symptomatic patients with the first episode of DVT with a positive predictive value of 97%. A normal proximal venous Doppler study excludes DVT with a negative predictive value of 98%. These studies are less reliable in diagnosing calf vein thrombosis. But calf vein thrombosis rarely results in pulmonary embolism. However, calf vein thrombosis may extend into the proximal veins from where it can embolize to the lungs. These studies can be used to detect such extension.

|More recently, color Doppler ultrasonography and real-time ultrasonography have been used to diagnosis DVT.[6] Duplex scanning, which combines ultrasound imaging and Doppler information, is now supplanting the former techniques. The duplex scan diagnoses symptomatic above-knee thrombosis with as high as 100% sensitivity and 98% specificity. Radiolabeled fibrinogen, which deposits in the area of clot, is highly sensitive in the diagnosis of DVT. However, this technique is expensive and is primarily useful as a research tool. D-dimer is a degradation product of cross-linked fibrin and is elevated in the presence of thrombus.[8] The absence of D-dimer provides strong evidence against thromboembolism. However the use of the D-dimer assay has not been widespread in the clinical diagnosis of DVT. Accurate assay of D-dimer takes several hours to perform and many hospitalized patients without thrombosis have elevated D-dimer levels.

|The venogram is the gold standard for the diagnosis of DVT. However, it is an invasive procedure associated with morbidity from such complications as dye-related renal failure, which may be especially problematic in patients with SCI who have an underlying renal insufficiency. The other tests described are so accurate that venography uncommonly has to be used.

Pulmonary Embolism [5, 6, 8]
|Pulmonary embolism is a major cause of death in patients with SCI. As is the case with many other conditions, the diagnosis of pulmonary embolism may be more difficult in patients with SCI than in ambulatory subjects. Unexplained symptoms of dyspnea, cough, hemoptysis, or apprehension should raise the suspicion of pulmonary embolism. Signs of pulmonary embolism include hemoptysis, cyanosis, hypotension, pleural friction rub, fever, loud pulmonic component of the second heart sound, or an S3 or S4 gallop. Hypoxemia is usually present. However, a patient with tetraplegia may not be able to sense chest pain, or may be dyspneic from some other cause.

|The ECG is abnormal in 70% of patients with pulmonary embolism. The most common abnormalities are sinus tachycardia (ST), non-specific ST, and T-wave changes. A small percent of patients have right atrial hypertrophy, right ventricular hypertrophy, right axis deviation with a large "S" wave in lead I and "Q" wave in lead III, or right bundle branch block. Arterial blood gases typically reveal respiratory alkalosis due to hyperventilation and hypoxemia. The chest X-ray is abnormal in 88% of patients with the findings of atelectasis, infiltrate, and pleural effusions. The chest X-ray is primarily useful to exclude other causes of chest pain, hemoptysis, and dyspnea. A totally normal chest X-ray in a patient with profound hypoxemia is highly suggestive of pulmonary embolism. However, abnormalities of blood gases may be difficult to interpret in patients with SCI, especially in those with tetraplegia with underlying pulmonary disease. If pulmonary embolism is suspected, a ventilation-perfusion scan or spiral computer-aided tomography (CT) scan should be performed. Areas that are ventilated but not perfused are likely sites of pulmonary embolism. A high-probability scan shows normal ventilation of areas that on perfusion scan are characterized by multiple defects that are wedge-shaped or segmental or that occur as concave defects on the lateral edges of the lung or on a pleural surface. A high-probability scan is usually adequate to make the diagnosis of pulmonary embolism. A negative perfusion scan excludes the diagnosis of pulmonary embolism.

|Spiral CT angiography is sensitive for the detection of a thrombus in the proximal pulmonary arteries, but not as sensitive in the segmental and subsegmental arteries.5 Helical or spiral CT angiography is 53% to 60% as sensitive and 81% to 97% as specific as pulmonary angiography for the detection of pulmonary thromboembolism. Pulmonary angiography is the gold standard for the diagnosis of pulmonary embolism. Pulmonary angiography should be performed when the ventilation/perfusion scan is of intermediate or low probability and embolism is still suspected, when there is increased risk of bleeding from anticoagulants or when the use of thrombolytic therapy or surgical treatment, such as embolectomy, is contemplated.

Treatment of Pulmonary Embolism and DVT [5,6,8]

|Because most pulmonary emboli arise from clots in the lower extremities the treatment of these two conditions is similar. The goal of anticoagulant therapy is to prevent further clot formation. Within 1 to 3 weeks, the clot will endothelialize and attach to the vessel wall, and the threat of dislodgement will be minimized. Heparin binds to and accelerates the ability of antithrombin III to inactivate thrombin, factor Xa, and factor IXa, thereby retarding thrombus formation. A loading dose of 80 units/kg of heparin is administered intravenously. A continuous infusion of heparin at an average rate of 18 units/kg/hour is then administered. Heparin is delivered at a rate sufficient to maintain the activated partial thromboplastin time (PTT) at 1.5 to 2.5 times the control. More recently low-molecular-weight heparins have been used in the treatment of pulmonary embolism and DVT. Low molecular weight heparins provide antithrombotic activity that is equal to or greater than unfractionated heparins with fewer hemorrhagic complications. They exhibit less protein binding than unfractionated heparin and have a longer plasma half-life and more predictable dose-response characteristics. They are administered subcutaneously twice a day in a dose that is determined by body weight and do not require monitoring of coagulation parameters. For example, enoxaparin is administered at a dose of 1 to 1.5 mg/kg twice a day. At the time heparin is begun, warfarin is started. Loading doses of warfarin are not required. The initial starting dose is usually 5 mg. This dose is continued for 2 to 4 days. Then the dose is adjusted to maintain a therapeutic international normalized ratio (INR). Warfarin inhibits synthesis of the vitamin K dependent factors II, VII, IX, and X. Warfarin also reduces levels of protein C and naturally occurring antithrombic protein. Protein C has a short half-life. Therefore, warfarin could temporarily induce a hypercoagulable state. For these reasons heparin is continued for 4 to 5 days after warfarin is started. An INR value between 2 and 3 is recommended for the treatment of venous thromboembolic disease. Oral anticoagulation should be continued for at least 3 months. It is possible that shorter periods of treatment are sufficient in some patients, but it is difficult to identify these patients. Anticoagulation beyond 3 months has not been shown to be beneficial. However, prolonged treatment is indicated when major underlying risk factors for a thrombotic event persist, such as a long immobilization, a hypercoagulable state (such as exists with an underlying malignancy), and recurrent DVT or pulmonary embolism.

|Thrombolytic treatment with tissue plasminogen activators, such as alteplase, is more effective than anticoagulation alone for the early restoration of the patency of a thrombosed vein.[8] Thrombolytic therapy may be indicated in patients with pulmonary embolism who are at high risk for death from the immediate consequence of obstruction of the pulmonary circulation. The major disadvantages of thrombolytic therapy compared with heparin are its greater cost and a significant increase in hemorrhagic complications such as intracranial hemorrhage. Patients with acute SCI have usually suffered major trauma, which often involves the brain. The use of thrombolytic agents in these patients is contraindicated.

|Occasionally anticoagulation is contraindicated in patients with SCI or patients have recurrent pulmonary embolism despite anticoagulation. In these circumstances, the vena cava can be interrupted to prevent clots from passing from the venous system to the lungs. Placement of the Greenfield filter, which is inserted into the vena cava via the right internal jugular vein or common femoral vein, is the most common method of interrupting the venal cava. Patients with SCI are at increased risk for complications from Greenfield filter placement. Balshi and colleagues found that in 13 instances in which a Greenfield filter was placed in patients with tetraplegia, 5 cases of abnormality in the filter were seen (distal migration, deformity, occlusion).[9] Laparotomy for bowel perforation was required in two of these patients. The occurrence of these complications correlated with the use of quad cough physical therapy. In patients with pulmonary compromise who require vigorous pulmonary toilet, vena caval interruption by some other means should be considered. However, total surgical interruption of the vena cava may result in dilation of retroperitoneal collateral veins, which are potential routes for large emboli.

|Most authors recommend anticoagulation for a longer time if a second episode of pulmonary embolism or DVT occurs (e.g., 12 months). A third episode may be an indication for lifelong anticoagulation.

Prevention of DVT

|The high incidence of DVT and pulmonary embolism during the first 3 months after SCI makes prophylaxis desirable. Pulmonary embolism can occur within 24 hours of a negative iodine 123-labelled fibrinogen scan and impedance plethysmography of the lower extremities. The clinical diagnosis of DVT is especially difficult in patients with SCI. Because the first pulmonary embolism is often fatal, prophylaxis is of critical importance.

|The Consortium for Spinal Cord Medicine has produced guidelines for the prevention of DVT in patients with SCI.[10] When possible, compression hose or pneumatic devices should be applied to the legs of patients for the first 2 weeks following injury. This prevents stasis. Anticoagulation with either low molecular weight heparin or adjusted-dose unfractionated heparin should be initiated within 72 hours after SCI provided there is no active bleeding or coagulopathy. Anticoagulants should be continued until discharge in patients with incomplete injuries, for 8 weeks in patients with uncomplicated complete motor injury, and for 12 weeks or until discharge from rehabilitation in those with complete motor injury and other risk factors, such as lower limb fractures or a history of thrombosis, cancer, obesity, or age over 70. Early mobilization and, if possible, exercise, should be initiated as soon as is medically feasible.

|Low-dose heparin (5,000 units) 2 to 3 times daily subcutaneously prevents thrombosis with little or no increase in risk of bleeding in ambulatory patients. However, a larger dose of heparin may be necessary to prevent DVT in patients with SCI. Green et al found that adjusting the heparin dose upward to prolong the activated partial thromboplastin time to 1.5 times the control level was superior to low-dose therapy in preventing DVT, but the larger dose of heparin increased the risk of hemorrhagic complications.[11] Low molecular weight heparin (e.g., enoxaparin given subcutaneously every 12 hours) or tinzaparin 3,500 units given once a day has been found to be superior to unfractionated heparin in the prevention of DVT in patients with SCI, with fewer hemorrhagic complications.[12] The work of Winemiller et al suggests that the prophylactic effect of heparin is the greatest during the first 14 days after injury, whereas the benefit from sequential-pneumatic compression continues to 6 weeks after injury.[13] Combining aspirin and dipyridamole with external calf compression may result in fewer thrombotic events than occur with calf compression alone.[6]

|Patients with acute SCI should be examined twice daily for signs of DVT, which include an increase in circumference of the calf or thigh, and increase in the venous pattern of collateral veins, pain or tenderness in the extremity or a low-grade fever. In symptomatic patients, ultrasonography of the extremity should be performed or ventilation/perfusion scanning in the case of suspected pulmonary embolism. Exercise, weight loss, cessation of smoking, and avoidance of constricting devices on the lower extremities will decrease the risk of DVT.

Conclusion

|Patients with SCI are at increased risk for DVT, especially during the acute phase. Doppler ultrasonography and ventilation/perfusion scans provide an accurate means of diagnosing DVT and pulmonary embolism. The treatment is anticoagulation with heparin and warfarin for the first 3 months. If anticoagulation is contraindicated, a Greenfield filter may be placed. DVT is prevented by early mobilization, calf compression, and heparin therapy.

References

1. Myllynen P, Kammonen M, Rakkanen P, et al. The blood FVIIIag/FVIIIc ratio as an early indicator of deep vein thrombosis during post-traumatic immobilization. *J Trauma* 1987;27:287.

2. Petaja J, Myllynen P, Rokkanen M, et al. Fibrinolysis and spinal cord injury. *Acta Chir Scand* 1989;155:241.

3. Vaziri N, Winer R, Alikhani S, et al. Antithrombin deficiency in end-stage renal disease associated with paraplegia. Effect of hemodialysis. *Arch Phys Med Rehab* 1985;66:307.

4. Myllynen P, Kammonen M, Rokkanen P, et al. Deep vein thrombosis and pulmonary embolism in patients with spinal cord injury. A comparison with nonparalyzed patients immobilized due to spinal fractures. *J Trauma* 1985;25:541.

5. Chestnut M, Prendergast T. Disorders of the pulmonary circulation. In: Tierney L, McPhee S, Papadakis M (Eds). *Current Medical Diagnosis and Treatment* (39th edition). Lange Medical Books McGraw Hill: New York, 2000; pp. 321-329.

6. Schmitt J, Midha M, McKenzie N. Medical Complications of Spinal Cord Disease. In: Young, R, Woolsey, R (Eds). *Diagnosis and Management of Disorders of the Spinal Cord*. WB Saunders: Philadelphia, 1995; pp. 297-316.

7. White RH, McGahan JP, Daschbach MM. Diagnosis of deep vein thrombosis using duplex ultrasound. *Ann Int Med* 1989;111:297.

8. Weinmann E, Salzman E. Deep vein thrombosis. *N Eng J Med* 1994;331:1630.

9. Balshi D, Contelmo N, Monzoian J. Complications of caval interruption by Greenfield filter for deep vein thrombosis in quadriplegics. *J Vasc Surg* 1989;9:558.

10. "Prevention of Thromboembolism" in Spinal Cord Injury Consortium for Spinal Cord Medicine. Clinical Practice Guidelines, 1999.

11. Green D, Lee M, Ito V. Fixed vs. adjusted dose heparin the prophylaxis of thromboembolism in spinal cord injury. *JAMA* 1988;260:1255.

12. Green D, Lee M, Lim A, et al. Prevention of thromboembolism after spinal cord injury with low molecular weight heparin. *Ann Int Med* 1990;113:571.

13. Winemiller M, Stolp-Smith K, Silverstein M, et al. Prevention of venous thromboembolism in patients with spinal cord injury: effects of sequential pneumatic compression and heparin. *J Spinal Cord Med*. 1999;22(3):182.

Addendum by the Editor

Deep vein thrombosis in patients with chronic SCI: The incidence of deep vein thrombosis (DVT) in acute SCI is high, varying statistics from 23% to 100%, yet it is very low in the chronic stage and does not seem to be higher than in the non-paralyzed population (0.8%).[1] The etiologic factors are different from those of the acute phase, especially with endothelial damage, hypercoagulopathy, and stasis. This may be explained by venous adaptation, muscle spasms and use of NSAIDs. In the chronic patient, DVT may develop de novo or may be a reactivation of an old phlebitis. The precipitating factors are usually trauma to soft tissue or bones and joints, or infections especially of the urinary tract, respiratory system, soft tissue, and bone (decubiti and osteomyelitis) — very rarely postoperatively (in our series of 7,000 surgeries, the incidence was 1:1000), more rarely with malignancy. It is usually manifested by edema of the lower extremity, color changes (congestion), low grade fever and tachycardia.[2-4] One should rule out fractures, ruptured muscle, especially with aspirin or non-steroidal anti-inflammatory drug (NSAID) intake, heterotopic ossification (HO), cellulitis, and compartment syndrome. However, these conditions may be associated with DVT, especially HO. Diagnosis is confirmed by noninvasive tests, fibrinogen uptake tests and phlebography. See above chapter for management.

|Pulmonary embolism is rare. Post phlebitis syndrome due to venous occlusion or insufficiency is noticed in about one third of the cases. It is manifested by refractory edema, pain, skin breakdown, stasis ulcers, and eczema. Sometimes recurrent DVT and even pulmonary embolus (PE) are noted. Management of these cases is difficult and entails physical therapy, elevation, massage, elastic bandage, and elastic stocking. Functional phlebography may be indicated for possible surgical intervention.

Superficial phlebitis: This occurs in varicose veins as phlebitis or thrombophlebitis. It may develop in cannulated veins especially when it is prolonged and with the use of strong chemicals. Occasionally, it is a manifestation of Buerger's disease, polycythemia, and polyarteritis. Rarely it is thrombophlebitis migrans, which may herald the presence of visceral cancer. Clinically the vein is inflamed and cordlike.

|Management: bed rest and leg elevation, elastic stocking, and NSAID therapy. If infection supervenes (as noticed by inflammation signs and leukocytosis), then antibiotics are prescribed. If thrombosis ascends quickly, emergency proximal ligation may be indicated. Embolism is very unusual. Rarely anticoagulants are indicated.

Suggested Reading

I. Lamb GC, Tomski MA, Kaufman J, et al. Is chronic spinal cord injury associated with increased risk of venous thromboembolism? *J Amer Paraplegia* 1993;16:153-156.

II. Stallman JS, Aisen PS, Aisen ML. Pulmonary embolism presenting as fever in spinal cord injury patients: Report of two cases and review of literature. *J Amer Paraplegia* 1993;16:157-159.

III. Cook AW, Lyons HA. Venous thromboembolism and other venous disease in the Tecumseh community health study. *Am J Med Sci* 1949;218:15-160.

IV. Kaufman JK, Kharti BO, Riendle P. Are patients with multiple sclerosis protected from thrombophlebitis and pulmonary embolism? *Chest* 1988;94:998-1001.

V. Attia J, Ray JE, et al. Deep vein thrombosis and its prevention in critically ill adults. *Arch of Internal Medicine* 2001;161, May 28:1268-1279.

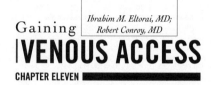

Gaining **Ibrahim M. Eltorai, MD; Robert Conroy, MD**

|VENOUS ACCESS

CHAPTER ELEVEN ▮▬▬▬▬▬▬▬

|In many patients with spinal cord injury (SCI), especially the chronic ones, the superficial veins of the extremities may have been all exhausted through many previous vein punctures, edema, and scars. Patients get infusions, transfusions, antibiotics, contrast media, blood tests, etc., and in some cases, illicit venipuncture. So it may be difficult and sometimes impossible to gain venous access, especially in emergencies for diagnostic and/or therapeutic procedures.

Phase one: What is the best way to gain venous access under normal conditions?

I. Perform venipuncture in good light.

II. If overlying hair is obscuring the veins, shave the area.

III. Know the anatomy of the superficial venous system and its surface marking.

IV. Distend the veins; do not overdistend because overdistended veins, especially in the elderly, tend to rupture after puncture.

V. Distension is achieved by the following:

A. Constricting band (rubber tourniquet) only to obstruct the venous outflow.

B. Inflating sphygmomanometer cuff inflated to about 80 mmHg.

C. Applying thumb pressure on the proximal part of the vein.

D. Relying on limb dependency.

E. Using warmth, hair dryer, warm pad, warm compresses, etc.

F. Gently tapping hand over the veins.

G. Repeating muscular exercise if feasible.

VI. If the vein is not visible, tapping over its course and feeling a fluid thrill with the other hand may identify it.

VII. Induce percutaneous anesthesia at the site of puncture, raising a bleb about ⅛ inch.

VIII. Avoid slipping of the vein by fixing it and straightening it by gently stretching the vein with overlying skin.

IX. Insert the needle almost vertically through the skin to be less painful. Align it over the vein and parallel to it, before gently depressing and pushing into it to pierce the superficial wall and enter the lumen and advancing it, seeing blood through the plastic sheath or through the metal needle shown in the syringe by aspiration.

X. For large slippery veins, try the puncture at the junction of the tributaries where the vein tends to be more stable.

XI. Release the tourniquet before any injection.

XII. In the wrist volar aspect and the antecubital site, palpate the radial artery and the brachial artery to avoid arterial puncture.

XIII. When you have to do venipuncture in the legs or feet, one routine is to check for the arterial circulation. In case of peripheral obliterative arterial disease, avoid venipuncture unless it is very necessary and watch closely for infiltration. Because patients with SCI have anesthetic skin, they may get extensive necrosis, which could result in amputation. Keep transparent dressing (Opsite) at the venipuncture site and observe the site regularly.

XIV. Avoid injecting contrast media in the leg that previously had deep vein thrombosis (DVT) to avoid reactivation.

XV. Avoid vasoactive medications in the lower extremity with peripheral vascular disease (PVD).

Phase two: Vyskocil et al,[2] describe several "tricks" for establishing venous access; the following is abstracted:

I. In edematous limbs: Elevate, massage the fluid upward, use Ace bandage until the fluid is cleared from the hand, put on the tourniquet, and do venipuncture. Then remove the tourniquet.

II. Apply 1 to 2 mg nitroglycerine ointment to the vein site.

III. Cuff inflation: Use sphygmomanometer cuff and inflate it to above systolic pressure for a few minutes, not exceeding 5. Hypoxia due to inflation will lead to vasodilation. Release pressure to just above the diastolic pressure. Try not to use this technique in patients with peripheral vascular disease.

IV. Vein detection by Doppler ultrasonography, especially in the external jugular vein. Both simple and sophisticated ultrasonographic machines (Dymax, Inc, Pittsburgh, PA) can be used with expert consultation. The Landry vein finder may be used. It consists of dual fiberoptic lights that transilluminate peripheral veins (Applied Biotech Products, Inc., 300 East Amedee, Scott, LA 70583).

Uncommon Venous Accesses

|Cut down on external jugular, distal saphenous, cephalic, or basilic veins. Employ femoral catheterization for emergency cases.

|When venous entry is impossible, one should use the central lines, such as Broviac or Hickman catheter, which have to be performed by the general or vascular surgeon. These techniques have now been replaced in most cases by the peripherally inserted central catheter (PICC) line.

Figure I **Placing a PICC Line With Fluoroscopic Guidance**

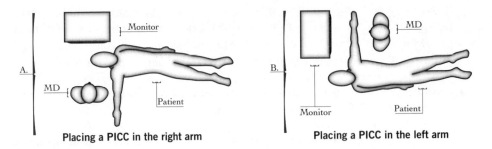

Placing a PICC in the right arm   Placing a PICC in the left arm

Placing a PICC line:

I. These lines are inserted in the upper arm for ease of the patient and convenience of use. The right or the left arm can be used. The PICC lines do not interfere with the use of the arms.

II. An IV is first started anywhere in the forearm or hand. A 21-gauge needle can be used. About 2 feet of extension tubing is attached to the IV needle.

III. The patient is placed on his back on a fluoroscopic table with the arm on an armboard, extended 90 degrees laterally and the palm upward.

IV. Contrast is hand injected into the IV. With a fluoroscope, the contrast is observed as it moves through the veins proximal to the elbow. The tip of a forceps is gently pushed against any large vein in the mid-position of the upper arm to mark the entry site of the PICC line into the vein. Do not push obliquely or from the side of the vein but directly from above. Any large vein in the upper arm is suitable for placing a PICC line. The vein can be medial, lateral, or in the middle of the arm. It can be immediately under the skin or 1, 2, or 3 inches deep, as long as it can be reached with an 18-gauge, single-wall puncture needle (the same needle used for puncture in arteriograms). With a felt pen, mark the skin at the tip of the forceps.

V. The wrist is gently taped to the armboard to keep the arm from rotating.

VI. Using sterile technique, the skin for 4 inches around the felt-pen mark is painted with Betadine and blotted dry with a towel. A Cook Inc. PICC line set #PICS-501-MPIS-NT 5.0FR can be used. Most of the time a 5F single-lumen PICC line is inserted. However, larger double-lumen PICC lines are available. The hole-drape from the PICC line set is stuck to the skin, with the felt pen mark in the middle of the hole. The arm is draped to the tip of the fingers.

VII. The fluoroscope is set on magnify mode and centered over the felt pen mark on the upper arm.

VIII. If the right arm is used for the PICC line, place a portable fluoroscopy TV monitor on the patient's left side opposite the patient's head. Stand on the patient's right side, cephalad to the outstretched arm. Face the TV monitor. In this way, your right hand is poised to puncture a vein and movements on the monitor screen are not "backward" (Figure IA).

|If the left arm is used for the PICC line, place a portable monitor on the patient's left side, cephalad to the patient's outstreched arm and facing caudad. Stand caudad to the outstretched arm. Face the monitor. Your right hand is in a position to easily puncture a vein and movements on the monitor screen are not "backward" (Figure IB).

IX. One or 2 ml of anesthetic is injected superficially under the skin at the site of the felt pen mark. Do no inject anesthetic around the vein or the vein will go into spasm.

X. Have an assistant hand-inject contrast through the IV in the arm. When the contrast comes into view on the TV monitor, puncture the skin with a 3-inch, 18-gauge artery puncture needle with a 5-cc syringe containing 2 ml of saline attached to the needle. Advance the needle until it indents the contrast-filled vein. Advance the needle through both walls of the vein. Aspirate gently on the syringe and slowly withdraw the needle. At the first signs of blood in the syringe, re-advance the needle 1 to 2 mm, remove the syringe and put the .018-inch guidewire supplied with the PICC set into the puncture needle. Do not push the wire out of the needle. Under fluoroscopic guidance, withdraw the needle 1 mm, then gently advance the wire 2 to 3 mm out the end of the needle. If the wire is in lumen of the vein, it will easily pass in a straight line into the vein. If the wire is not in the vein, the wire will quickly bend away from the confines of the vein. If the wire is not in the vein, pull the wire back into the needle, withdraw the needle an additional 1 mm, and gently re-advance the wire. Continue this maneuver of the needle withdrawal and wire advancement until the wire is in the lumen of the vein.

XI. Advance the wire into the superior vena cava using fluoroscopic guidance to avoid passing the wire into tributaries.

XII. Remove the needle and place the dilator-sheath combination from PICC set over the wire into the vein. Position the tip of the wire where the tip of the catheter will be positioned. Put a clamp on the wire where it comes off the dilator.

XIII. Remove the guidewire, with the clamp attached, from the dilator. Cut the PICC line to the same length as the distance from the tip of the guidewire to the attached clamp.

XIV. Place the stiffener wire into the PICC line. Remove the dilator from the sheath, and put the PICC line + wire through the sheath into the superior vena cava. Observe the advance of the PICC line + wire with fluoroscope to ensure the wire does not enter a tributary. Remove the peel-stiffening wire from the PICC line. Put a valve on the end of the PICC line. Inject 2 to 3 ml of heparin solution into the PICC line and suture the PICC line to the skin (Figure II).

Figure II **Inserted PICC Line**

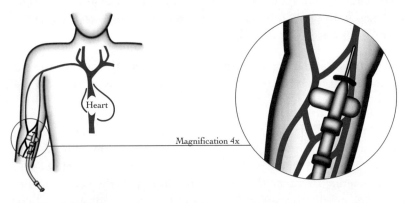

Heart

Magnification 4x

Venous Access Complications

I. Hematoma: manifested by swelling and discoloration. The line should be discontinued, direct pressure should be applied, and the limb should be elevated.

II. Extravasation of IV fluids due to misplacement or displacement of the cannula into the sheath or perivascular tissue of the vessel or through its side or back wall. In patients with SCI, pain is not perceived in lower extremity veins. Irritant substances such as KCl, norepinephrine, vancomycin, and chemotherapeutics lead to sloughing and, in a limb with peripheral arterial disease—especially diabetes, may lead to an amputation or at least debridement followed by skin grafting.[4]

III. Phlebitis: [5-8]

    A. Chemical phlebitis, e.g., with KCl, vancomycin, hypertonic saline or glucose, pentothal, or acidic infusions are preventable by dilution and flushing with normal saline or with 5 cc of 4.2% NaHCO3 to neutralize acidic fluids.

    B. Septic phlebitis usually occurs in catheters left in for weeks. It is manifested by pain, tenderness, induration, pyrexia, and sometimes toxemia. The catheter should be removed and superficial phlebectomy done plus antibiotic therapy.

IV. Central lines are liable to:

    A. Catheter sepsis, thrombosis, and embolism.

    B. Catheter or guidewire embolus.

    C. Superior vena caval or cardiac perforation.

    D. Pneumothorax.

    E. Air embolism.

    F. Malplacements.

    G. Thoracic duct injury when the catheter is inserted into the left side.

|These are rare complications and should be managed by a vascular surgeon and interventional radiologist and should be prevented.

Conclusion

|In patients with SCI, venous access is frequently hard to find due to repeated vein puncture for investigation or therapies. The standard technique is described with helpful hints.

|When it is impossible to find access, especially if the patient is on prolonged intravenous therapy, central line is the method of choice. Broviac or Hickman catheters are replaced by peripherally inserted central catheter (PICC) line. The method is described and it has to be done by an interventional radiologist.

References

1. Kirk RM. *Basic Surgical Techniques, Third edition*. Churchill Livingstone: Edinburgh, London, Melbourne & New York, 1989:pp. 94-06.

2. Vyskocil JJ, Kruse JD, Wilson RF. Alternating techniques for gaining venous access. *J Critical Illness* 1993;8(3):435-442.

3. Vyskocil JJ, Kruse JD, Wilson RF. Techniques in vascular access when venous entry is impossible. *J Critical Illness* 1993;8(4):539-545.

4. James EC, Carry Robert J, Perry John F. *Principles of Basic Surgical Practice*. Hanley and Belfus Inc.: Philadelphia; C.V. Mosby: St Louis, Toronto, London, 1987:pp. 485-87.

5. Paz-Fumagalli R, Miller YA, Russell BA, et al. Impact of peripherally inserted central catheter on phlebitic complications of peripheral intravenous therapy. *Spinal Cord Med* 1997;20(3):341-344.

6. Cardella JF, Fox PS, Lawler JB. Interventional radiologic placement of peripherally inserted catheters. *J Vasc Interventional Radiol* 1993;4:653-660.

7. Cardella JF, Cardella K, Bacci N, et al. Cumulative experience with 1,273 peripherally inserted central catheters at a single institution. *J Vasc Interventional Radiol* 1996;7:5-13.

8. Maki DG. Infections due to infusion therapy. In: Bennett JV, Brachman PS (Eds). *Hospital infections*. Little, Brown and Company: Boston, 1992:pp. 849-898.

Acute
|ARTERIAL OCCLUSION
of the Lower Extremities

Ibrahim M. Eltorai, MD;
Bok Y. Lee, MD, FACS

CHAPTER TWELVE

|With the increasing longevity of patients with spinal cord injury (SCI), there is increasing prevalence of peripheral arterial disease. Modern non-invasive testing technology has made it possible to detect more peripheral arterial disease cases. Cardiovascular disorders in this population, such as coronary artery disease, autonomic dysreflexia, hypertension, hypotension, and deep venous thrombosis, have received much attention in research but peripheral arterial disease has not. These arterial occlusive diseases are frequently missed by the clinician partly because of lack of pain sensation, especially that of intermittent claudication, and partly due to the absence of symptoms.

Predisposing Factors

I. Disorders of carbohydrate metabolism and impaired glucose tolerance lead to diabetes mellitus.[1,2] According to the World Health Organization criteria, the incidence of diabetes mellitus in the SCI population was 22% compared to 6% in the general population. The resulting hyperglycemia will alter the arterial wall metabolism with the accumulation of chemical products.

II. Dyslipidemia: The lowering of high density lipoprotein (HDL) cholesterol in patients with SCI was 24% to 40%, compared to 10% in ambulatory patients.[1,2] This is attributed to lack of mobility, obesity, and a high intake of fatty and high calorie foods, all of which increases the serum triglycerides.

III. Spasticity and contractures may mechanically impede the arterial circulation.

IV. Nicotine addiction: The role of cigarette smoking is not entirely clear. By producing hypoxia, it may lower the HDL and raise the low density lipoprotein (LDL), thus injuring the endothelium. This may also stimulate proliferation of the arterial smooth muscle and combined with nicotine vasoconstriction there is increased lysomal activity permitting greater LDL accumulation in the arterial wall.[3] The toxic effects of other smoke components are not clearly known.[3]

V. Other factors acting with patients with SCI have not been studied: elevated fibrinogen level, elevated iron level, elevated uric acid, hypothyroidism, oxidation stress, hypertension, hyperhemoxysternemia, psychodynamic factors, and genetic predisposition. These may be important factors especially in the development of premature peripheral atherogenesis before the age of 50.

|In general, atherosclerosis has a higher incidence in patients with SCI as evidenced by a higher incidence of coronary heart disease, Gordon et al found a two-fold risk of abdominal aortic aneurysm in patients with SCI as compared with ambulatory patients.[4-7] Similarly, we encountered several cases of Leriche's syndrome in lower lumbar injuries (unpublished personal experience presented to APS 1990).[8]

VI. Incidence of peripheral vascular disease (PVD) of the lower extremities in patients with SCI:

|Routine exams for PVD in patients with SCI are not well documented and frequently missing from the patient's history and physical examination. Wythe et al conducted a study on 50 patients with SCI, ages 28 to 82, with different levels of injury. All of these were chronic cases and various factors were analyzed with the conclusion that PVD is more predominant in patients with SCI with a rate of 20% than in ambulatory patients with a rate from 5% to 10%. The incidence is increasing with age, the duration of SCI, diabetes mellitus, dyslipidemia, hypertension, cigarette smoking, and large joint contractures with significant joint deformity. Also, the higher the level of injury, the higher the incidence of PVD.[8]

Clinical Picture

|As mentioned previously, detection of PVD in patients with SCI is difficult and is often overseen. For this purpose we will describe two forms: quiescent (Forme masquee) and acute (Forme ouverte).

I. The quiescent form can be detected only by paying attention to the vasculature of the lower extremities by physical examination, clinically with non-invasive testing, especially in patients who have the risk factors mentioned previously. Some patients will present non-healing decubitus ulcers or frequent surgical failures.

II. The acute form is usually due to a thrombosis developing in the atherosclerotic arteries at different levels. Frequent causes are soft tissue trauma, thermal injuries, acute infection or a fracture; viz., supracondylar femoral fracture, use of circular casts, infiltration of chemicals (especially vancomycin given in leg veins), compartment syndromes anterior tibial or adductor canal) often with hematomata, sepsis with shock or volume depletion, congestive heart failure, or malignancy. We encountered (unpublished) a case of bilateral gangrene due to phlegmasia cerulea from metastatic pulmonary carcinoma. Another case with anterior tibial compartment compression from neglected IV infusion subfascially in the leg.

|Acute arterial occlusion may result from emboli due to myocardial infarction, atrial fibrillation, prosthetic heart valve, or aortoiliac or femoral atherosclerotic lesion. Rarely is it due to bacterial endocarditis.

Diagnosis—Quiescent Form

|The quiescent form requires a timely diagnosis, especially in patients with risk factors. The tibials, popliteal, or femoral vessels should undergo a complete vascular exam with the use of non-invasive modalities. The extremity will show decreased or absent pulse by palpation or by ultrasound probe, the ankle brachial index is low (depending on the degree of ischemia), trophic change, loss of hair, decreased temperature, discoloration (pallor or congestion), non-healing pressure ulcer especially on the heel and the malleoli, epidermophytosis, or onychomycosis. A note of caution: Patients with cold blue feet, possibly with a history of deep vein thrombosis (DVT), edema, and stasis ulceration may have venostasis from prolonged sitting time in a wheelchair. Elevation and bed rest may resolve these and should not be confused with acute arterial occlusion. Associated coronary vascular disease may be detected. Routine abdominal ultrasound may show an aneurysm or aortic bifurcation narrowing.

Diagnosis—Acute Form

|The acute form presents acute ischemia either thrombotic or embolic. Other forms of vascular disease are rarely encountered, e.g., Bueger's thromboangiitis obliterans and other kinds of vasculitis. There is absence of pulse, the limb is cold, color changes from pallor to cyanosis, marble appearance, blisters, edema, necrotic patches, dry gangrene or wet gangrene in diabetics.[9]

Clinical diagnosis: Non-invasive laboratory tests.[9-13]

    I. Ankle Brachial Index — below 0.4 is serious.

    II. Duplex ultra-sonography, Doppler color flow, imaging for measurement of the blood vessel and blood flow.

    III. Transcutaneous PO_2 – below 40.0 is critical.

    IV. Other tests (rarely needed):

        A. Impedance plethysmography.

        B. Toe index systolic pressure versus finger pressure.

        C. Digital imaging.

    V. Invasive tests (when intervention is needed):

        A. Angiography by the Sedlinger technique to define the level and degree of occlusion; collateral circulation and runoff to decide which therapy is needed.

        B. Catheter-based technique produces images of the vascular lumen with digital imaging.[13]

    VI. Magnetic resonance imaging with contrast.

    VII. Intravascular sonography describes vascular characteristic and morphology.

Management
Quiescent form:

I. Cessation of any forms of tobacco (cigarette, cigar, pipe, snuff, chew, etc.).

II. Lipid lowering by diet and pharmacotherapy.

III. Antiplatelet agents, i.e., aspirin, clopidogrel, Plavix, Ticlid, dipyridamole.

IV. Prostaglandin E or calcium channel blockers. [5]

V. Rheologic agents: pentoxifylline (Trental), ketanserin.

VI. Cilostazol is a new phosphodiesterase inhibitor that suppresses platelet aggregation and also acts as a direct arterial vasodilator.

|In the absence of manifest ischemic lesions, such as ulcers or non-healing wounds, or ischemic flaps, surgery is usually not indicated, but periodic and close follow-ups are necessary. The precipitating factors for acute occlusion should be treated and prevented. Avoid pressure sores, trauma, thermal or hypothermic injuries, and fungus infections. The patient should not wear tight-fitting shoes and braces. Local hygiene of the feet, especially in diabetes, is important. The patient or his/her caregiver should be alert to cuts, sores, or color changes to the feet and report them to a physician. A podiatrist should be seen for care of the feet including toenails and calluses. Other experimental drugs, such as growth factors and gene therapy, are in the experimental stage and are not applicable to SCI cases at this time. Conservative treatment is indicated for small pressure ulcers, ischemic ulcers, localized patches of gangrenous skin, or dry gangrene of one or more toes.[14]

Acute form: The concept of amputation because the limb is paralyzed was adopted for decades. Today, with the current technology, many limbs may be saved as long as tissue ischemia is not very advanced and revascularization is possible and limb salvage can be achieved. Limb salvage can be achieved in some cases by:

I. Pharmacotherapy:

A. Heparinization.

B. Fibrinolysis may be produced through an arterial catheter using Streptokinase or tissue plasminogen activator (TPA). These should be avoided in patients with coagulopathies, such as hepatic, renal, cardiac, or cerebral lesions. Urokinase has been discontinued by the FDA. Reteplase seems to hold greater promise for PVD.[15-20]

II. Surgery:

A. Endovascular procedures.[21-23]

i. Angioplasty.

ii. Laser endarterectomy.

iii. Stent placement.

iv. Embolectomy in cases of an embolism.

B. Bypass surgeries. These are done for salvageable limbs especially when paralysis is incomplete. It is contraindicated in case of progressive ischemia. The surgeries depend on:

i. The level and degree of the occlusion.

ii. More needed when there is residual function in the limb.

iii. May be needed when there are large pressure ulcers refractory to flap reconstruction or in cases of a non-healing of amputation stump

iv. The techniques have to be decided by the vascular surgeon after angiography.

v. Aortoiliac occlusion may require aortofemoral bypass.

vi. In high-risk patients or those with abdominal scars or suprapubic cystostomy, or colostomy, axillofemoral bypass is an alternative.

vii. Superficial femoral occlusions do well with endovascular techniques or femoropopliteal bypass.[6,24]

viii. Tibial occlusions are difficult and endovascular techniques are of limited usefulness.

III. Lumbar sympathetectomy in patients with digital gangrene not amenable to direct arterial procedures is beneficial. Lee and Thoden reported a 5-year cumulative limb salvage rate of 71% and a toe salvage rate of 51%.[26] These results are mainly in ambulatory patients; they are expected to be different in patients with SCI with cord transection. The use of predictive criteria for proper patient selection is invaluable in preventing overuse of sympathectomy.

IV. Amputation is indicated when ischemia is irreversible and tissue death has occurred, more so when there is sepsis in diabetics. The level of amputation is determined by the level of arterial occlusion, the collateral circulation, the degree of ischemia, and the degree of infection. Amputation may also be done in cases where revascularization is not possible due to general health problems. Transcutaneous PO_2 readings may help as an indicator of level choice. Diabetic feet need special consideration depending on the disease itself and its complications.[31]

V. Adjunctive therapy, viz., hyperbaric oxygen treatment (HBO_2) with impaired circulation there is tissue hypoxia.[27] HBO_2 has been found to elevate tissue oxygen levels thereby enhancing white cell function to fight infection and improving wound capacity for healing. It helps control anaerobic and microaerophilic bacteria. It is an adjunctive therapy for anaerobic infections postoperatively, when the result of revascularization is not optimum, and for impaired amputation flap circulation. The therapy is still controversial, but many studies are being done to assess its effects on ischemic reperfusion injuries and the microcirculation. It was of some benefit in arterial trauma, crush injuries, revision of vascularization procedures, ischemic flaps, and limb replantation.[28-30] More controlled studies are needed.

Conclusion

|Peripheral vascular disease (PVD) is common in the lower extremities of patients with SCI. This is due to immobility, spasticity, contractures, dyslipidemia, and diabetes mellitus. Excess smoking is an additional factor. PVD is manifested in two ways—the chronic form, which may not be detected clinically except in association with delayed or non-healing pressure ulcers or compromised flap circulation. It is frequently unthought of by the clinician due to analgesia and the absence of claudication. Some cases may develop acute ischemia, mainly thrombotic, precipitated by trauma, fracture, sepsis, volume depletion, heart failure, malignancy, and compartment syndromes.

|Management of the acute form should follow the same regimen for ambulatory patients, viz., medical and surgical intervention if gangrene has not proceeded. Endovascular procedures and bypasses can lead to salvage of the extremity. Amputation should be considered when gangrene has incurred or when the ischemic changes are irreversible or revascularization is impossible.

|The preceding is merely an outline for the general practitioner or the paraplegist. Consultation with specialists is always recommended.

References

1. Bauman WA, Kahn NN, Grimm DR, Spungen AM. Risk factors for artherogenesis and cardiovascular autonomic functions in persons with spinal cord injury. *Spinal Cord* 1999;37:601-616.

2. Bauman WA. Carbohydrate and lipid metabolism after spinal cord injury. *T Spinal Cord Inj Rehab* 1997;2(4):1-22.

3. Spungen RM et al. Prevalence of cigarette smoking in a group of male veterans with chronic spinal cord injury. *Mil Med* 1995;160:303-311.

4. Arrowood JA, Monhanty PK, Thames, MD. Cardiovascular problems in the spinal cord injured. *Medical Complications of Spinal Cord Injury*. Hanley and Belfus: Philadelphia, 1987; pp. 443-456.

5. Whiteneck G, Charlifue S, Gerhart K, et al. Aging with spinal cord injury. *The Cardiovascular System*. Demos Publication: New York, 1993; pp. 73-93.

6. Yookoo DM, Kronn, ML, Lewis VI et al. Peripheral vascular disease in spinal cord injury patients. *Ann Plas Surg* 1996;37(5):495-499.

7. Gordon I, et al. Spinal cord injury increases the risk of abdominal aortic aneurysm. *Am Surg* 1996;62(3):249-262.

8. Whythe W, Bonebakker DC, Eltorai IM, et al. Clinical vascular assessment in the spinal cord injury patient. A preliminary report presented to the American Paraplegia Society annual meeting 1990; Unpublished. Available from Eltorai by request.

9. James EC, Carry RJ, Perry JF. Acute arterial occlusion. In: *Principles of Basic Surgical Practice 1987*. Hanley and Belfus: Philadelphia, 1987; pp. 428-434.

10. Kit BP, Vacek JL, Savina L. Non-invasive approaches to peripheral vascular disease. *Post Grad Med* 1999;(3);52-64.

11. Fronek A, Coel M, Berstein EF. Quantitative ultrasonograph studies of lower extremity flow velocities in health and disease. *Circulation* 1996;53(6);957-960.

12. Bernstein EF. *Non-invasive diagnostic techniques in vascular disease*. C.V. Mosby: St. Louis, 1985.

13. Lips DL, Vasec JL. Catheter based methods for managing peripheral vascular disease. *Postgrad Med* 1999;106(3):69-82.

14. Lavery LA, Kenrick, DJ. Clinics in podiatric medicine and surgery. *Diabetic Foot* 1995: 12(1): 1-17.

15. Blaisdell FW, Steele M, Allen RE. Management of acute lower extremity arterial ischemia due to embolism and thrombosis. *Surgery* 1976;84:822-824.

16. Dardik H, Sussman BC, Kahn M, et al. Lysis of arterial clot by intravenous or intra-arterial administration of Streptokinase. *Surg Gyn & Ob* 1984;158: 137-140.

17. Taylor LM Jr, Porter JM, Bauer AM, et al. Intra-arterial Streptokinase infusion for acute popliteal and tibial artery occlusion. *Am J Surg* 1984;147:583-588.

18. Quriel K, Vieth FJ, Sasahara A. Thrombolysis or peripheral arterial surgery (TOPAS) investigators. A comparison of recombitant urokinase with vascular surgery as initial treatment for acute arterial occlusion of the legs. *N Eng J Med* 1998:338(16):1105-11.

19. McNamara TO. From New Pharmacologic Therapies in the Treatment of Peripheral Vascular Disease. Presented during the 11th Annual Symposium, Transcatheter Cardiovascvular Therapeutics: Washington. D.C.: September 22-26, 1999.

20. A Medi-Fax™ report from data presented at the 11th Annual Symposium, Transcatheter Cardiovascvular Therapeutics: Pharmacologic Therapies in the Treatment of Peripheral Vascular Disease Washington. D.C.: September 22-26, 1999.

21. James EC, Carry RJ, Perry, JF. Transilluminar angioplasty. In: *Principles of Basic Surgical Practice 1987*. Hanley and Belfus: Philadelphia:; pp. 435-443.

22. Gallino A, Mahler F, Probst P. Percutaneous angioplasty of the arteries of the lower limbs: a five–year follow-up. *Circulation* 1984;70:619-623.

23. Ginther RW, Vorwerk D, Bohndorf K, et al. Iliac and femoral artery stenoses and occlusions: treatments with intravascular stents. *Radiology* 1989;172(3):725-730.

24. Lee BY, Guerra J. Axillo-femoral bypass graft in a spinal cord injured patient with impending gangrene. *J Am Par Soc* 1994;17(4):171-176.

25. Dalman RI, Harris EJ, Walker MT, Perkash I. Limbs salvage surgery in spinal cord injury patients. *Ann Vas Surg* 1998;12(1):60-64.

26. Lee BY, Thoden WR. The role of sympathectomy in peripheral vascular surgery. *Practice of Surgery*, HS Goldsmith Medical Department. Harper and Row Publishers: Philadelphia, 1981; pp. 1-34.

27. Lee BY, Ostrander LE, Karmaker M, et al. Non-invasive quantification of muscle oxygen in subjects with and without claudication. *J Rehab Res Devel* 1997;34(1):44-51.

28. Zamboni WA. The microcirculation and ischemic reperfusion. In: *Basic Mechanisms of Hyperbaric Oxygen in Hyperbaric Medicine Practice* Kindwall EP. Best Publishing Company: Flagstaff, AZ, 1997; pp. 561-564.

29. Bergofsky EH, Bertrum R. Response of regional circulation to hypoxia. *J App Physiology* 1966;2:567.

30. Jain KK. Hyperbaric Oxygen Therapy in Cardiovascular Disease. In: *Hyperbaric Medicine*. Hogrefe and Huber, Publishers: Seattle, Toronto, 1996; pp. 317-341.

|SPASTICITY | Robert M. Woolsey, MD

and Spasms Associated With Spinal Cord Disorders
CHAPTER THIRTEEN

|Disruption of the spinal cord interrupts tracts from the cerebral cortex and from the brain stem that inhibit various spinal reflexes. One result of this loss of inhibition is the emergence of spasticity and spasms.

<u>Figure I</u> **Pathophysiology: Reflex Pathways From Receptor Through Spinal Cord to Muscle**

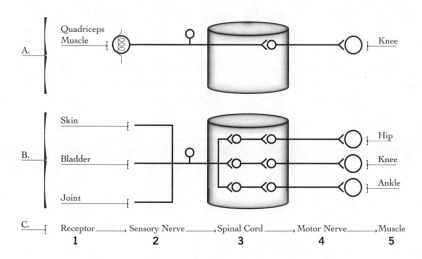

|Spasticity is a state of increased muscle tone resulting from hyperactivity of the stretch reflex (Figure IA). This reflex originates from the muscle spindle, which is the stretch receptor. When the receptor is activated, neural impulses are generated that pass through axons within a peripheral nerve. Upon reaching the spinal cord, these axons synapse directly upon anterior horn cells, the axons of which pass back through a peripheral nerve to the muscle from which the stimulus was generated, producing contraction of that muscle. This reflex is best illustrated by the "tendon jerk" elicited during the neurological examination. When anterior horn cells are continuously active, due to loss of inhibitory influences, continuous muscle contraction occurs, resulting in spasticity.[1]

|Although spasticity is almost universally present in patients with spinal cord disorders, it is rarely a clinical problem and may actually be a useful phenomenon that enables a patient to stand on a paralyzed leg. Occasionally, spasticity may be so severe that it impedes movement of a weak extremity or holds an extremity in an inconvenient position, as when bilateral thigh adductor spasticity interferes with catheter care or sexual function.

|Spasms are intermittent contractions of a group of synergistic muscles, such as all of the lower extremity flexors or extensors (Figure IB).[2] This reflex originates from receptors in a number of body structures including skin, muscle, bone, bladder, and gastrointestinal tract. When stimulated, these receptors generate an action potential that passes through axons in a peripheral nerve to the spinal cord. When these axons pass into the spinal cord, they branch into multiple divisions that travel up and down the spinal cord in a white matter tract that caps the gray matter of the dorsal horn (Lissauer's tract), from which they enter the dorsal horn gray matter and make contact with anterior horn cells innervating a group of synergistic muscles, i.e., hip flexors, knee flexors, and ankle dorsiflexors. When these receptors are activated by stimuli from such sources as pressure sores, bladder infection, fractures, etc., troublesome flexor or extensor spasms may result. If the stimulation is intense, more or less continuous spasms result, holding the legs in a flexion or extension position resembling a contracture. Contracture may in fact result if the spasms are not managed. Less frequent spasms may significantly interfere with activities of daily living, such as wheelchair transfers.

Treatment

|When treating spasticity or spasms, the opportunity exists to intervene at multiple sites (Figure IC) along the reflex pathway, mediating the abnormal muscle activity.[3]

I. Decreasing receptor stimulation is especially helpful in controlling spasms. Managing pressure sores, bladder infections, etc., will frequently abolish or at least markedly diminish spasms. Spasticity cannot usually be treated at the receptor level.

II. The reflex pathway for spasticity or spasms can be interrupted by surgical, chemical, or radio frequency destruction of a peripheral nerve or nerve root (rhizotomy). This is rarely done, as other, less complicated therapy is usually effective.

III. Both spasticity and spasms can be treated pharmacologically at the spinal cord level by suppressing the transmission stimuli entering the dorsal horn to the motor neurons of the anterior horn. Diazepam (Valium) enhances the effect of the inhibitory neurotransmitter GABA. Usually, daily doses of 20 mg or more are required. Baclofen (Lioresal) causes membrane hyperpolarization of axons in the reflex pathway and may have other mechanisms of action as well. Effective doses of baclofen range from 80 to 160 mg daily. Tizanidine (Zanaflex) prevents the release of excitatory neurotransmitters and may facilitate the action of the inhibitory neurotransmitter glycine. There is a general consensus that baclofen, because of its effectiveness and tolerable side effects, is the preferred drug. However, because the agents all act by somewhat different mechanisms, they may be used together in difficult cases.

|In cases of severe lower extremity spasticity or spasms in which oral medication is ineffective or cannot be tolerated, implantation of a baclofen pump should be considered.[4] A programmable pump is implanted subcutaneously in the abdominal wall. An attached catheter is placed into the spinal subarachnoid space near the conus medullaris, where baclofen can be delivered at a constant rate. Because the effective intrathecal dose of baclofen is about 1% of the oral dose, much higher doses can be delivered to the site of action by the pump than is possible with oral dosing. The pump can be refilled by transcutaneous injection as needed, usually about every 3 months. The procedure is highly effective, but expensive.

|In the past, the reflex pathway was surgically interrupted within the spinal cord by performing the so-called "T-myelotomy," but this has been superceded by pharmacological management.

IV. The reflex pathway can also be interrupted by destruction of the axon of the anterior horn cell. Obturator neurectomy was widely done in the past to control lower extremity adductor spasticity. The terminal portion of the axon can be destroyed by injecting motor points with phenol. More recently, botulinum toxin (Botox) has been injected into hypertonic muscles. This toxin prevents the release of acetylcholine from nerve terminals. Though effective, this treatment is very expensive and the duration of relief is only 3 to 6 months.

V. Dantrolene sodium (Dantrium) prevents calcium release from the endoplasmic reticulum of muscle, which is a necessary antecedent for muscle contraction. However, this drug affects spastic and normal muscles to an equal degree so that a patient with lower-level quadriplegia or paraplegia might lose upper extremity strength needed for wheelchair propulsion and transfers. Dantrolene also carries a substantial risk of toxic hepatitis.

VI. Tendonotomy of the iliopsoas or quadriceps muscles to control contractures and spasms of the hip or knee flexor muscles has been done in the past.[5] Muscle contraction is rendered ineffective because the muscle is no longer attached to bone. These procedures are now rarely done.

Conclusion

|Spasticity and spasms can be controlled in many ways. Techniques that are complex, require major surgery, or involve destruction of nerves or muscles are rarely needed. Spasms can frequently be managed simply by decreasing receptor stimulation by pressure sores or bladder infection. In almost all patients with spasticity or spasms, it is possible to pharmacologically suppress the responsible reflex pathway using baclofen, diazepam, tizanidine, or a combination of these drugs. In an occasional case, a baclofen pump might be useful.

References

1. Young RR, Delwaide PJ. Spasticity. *N Eng J Med* 1981;304:28-33, 96-99.

2. Guttmann L. *Spinal Cord Injuries Comprehensive Management and Research.* Ed. 2, Blackwell Scientific Publications: Oxford, 1973, pp. 515-529.

3. Gracies JM, Elovic E, McGuire J, Simpson D. Traditional pharmacological treatments for spasticity: Part I: Local treatments, Part II: General and regional treatments. *Muscle Nerve* 1997;20(suppl 6):S61-120.

4. Ordia JI, Fischer E, Adamski E, Spatz EL. Chronic intrathecal delivery of baclofen by a programmable pump for the treatment of spasticity. *J Neurosurg* 1996;86:452-456.

5. Eltorai I, Montroy R. Muscle release in the management of spasticity in spinal cord injury. *Paraplegia* 1990;28:433-440.

Acute and Chronic

|PAIN
Robert M. Woolsey, MD

With Spinal Cord Disorders
CHAPTER FOURTEEN ████████████████

|Pain is a common problem in patients with spinal cord disorders. Two-thirds of patients with spinal cord injury (SCI) have some type of pain and about one-fifth of these patients rate their pain as being so severe that it is the major factor limiting their quality of life.

|Pain associated with SCI may be of several types, each of which has a distinct neurological mechanism. Successful treatment depends upon accurate identification of the mechanism involved, which in turn depends upon understanding the anatomical and physiological features of the neural pathways involved in pain perception. These will be briefly reviewed (Figure I).

Figure | **Peripheral and Central Ascending and Descending Pathways Concerned With Pain**

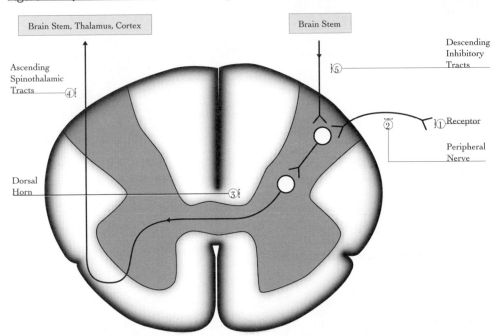

|Under normal circumstances, pain perception begins at the receptor (1). Pain receptors are the peripheral terminals of axons whose cell bodies are in the dorsal root ganglion. Deforming the axon will depolarize it, causing generation of an action potential directed toward the spinal cord. Also, most painful stimuli injure tissue, which causes the production of "algesic substances" such as potassium ions, bradykinin, prostaglandin, etc. These algesic substances depolarize pain receptors, causing the generation of action potentials. The axons conveying pain sensation pass from the receptor to the spinal cord through a peripheral nerve (2). When the pain axon arrives as the spinal cord, it enters the gray matter of the dorsal horn (3) where it will synapse with a transmission cell, the axon of which will convey the pain impulse to the brain or brain stem. The dorsal horn is more than a simple relay center. It is a complex neural processing center in which pain sensation may be facilitated or inhibited by other neurons of that spinal segment, by spinal segments above or below it, or by neurons of the brain or brain stem. The axon of the transmission cell crosses to the ventrolateral white matter of the opposite side and then ascends in the spinothalamic tract to terminate reticular formation in the brain stem or in the thalamus. Secondary fibers from the thalamus pass to the sensory cortex of the cerebral hemisphere. As previously stated, neurons from various levels of the brain stem send axons to the dorsal horn of the spinal cord where they can inhibit or facilitate transmission of pain sensation.

Types of Pain

|Pain can be broadly classified into two fundamental varieties: nociceptive pain and neuropathic pain.[1] Nociceptive pain is "normal pain" that is perceived in the manner outlined in the preceding paragraph, i.e., a noxious stimulus activates a pain receptor, which generates an action potential that proceeds through the peripheral and central pain pathways to the brain where it is recognized as a painful sensation. Acute or chronic nociceptive pain is usually "aching" in quality, variable in intensity from mild to severe, and is localized to the site from which it originates.

|Neuropathic pain, on the other hand, originates from damage to the transmission system itself. A peripheral nerve generates action potentials from an area of damage, which then pass through the remaining peripheral and central pain pathways to the brain where they are perceived in the distribution served by the damaged nerve, i.e., damage to the ulnar nerve at the elbow causes pain in the ring and little finger of the hand. This is "peripheral neuropathic pain." Likewise, if the pain pathways within the brain or spinal cord are damaged, pain may be perceived in both legs or on one entire side of the body. This is "central neuropathic pain."

|Because neuropathic pain is generated from a damaged area of the sensory pathways, it is usually associated with other abnormalities, such as sensory loss and hypersensitivity (hyperalgesia) in the painful area. In addition, non-painful stimuli may be perceived as painful (allodynia). Such findings are important indicators that a particular pain is neuropathic in origin. Neuropathic pain frequently has a "burning," "tingling," or "shooting" quality and is usually not as well localized as nociceptive pain.

|Patients with SCI may have any or all of these types of pain.[2] Pain must be correctly identified to be effectively treated because drug therapy is targeted at the mechanism by which pain is generated. With a few exceptions, drugs useful in treating nociceptive pain are not very helpful in the management of neuropathic pain and vice versa.

|Nociceptive pain in patients with SCI usually arises from damage to the bones and/or ligaments of the vertebral column resulting from fractures, infection, arthritis, neoplasm, etc. The pain is usually localized mainly to the involved vertebrae and aggravated by pressing upon or moving the involved area.

|Peripheral neuropathic pain in patients with SCI originates from damage to nerve roots (or dorsal root ganglia) by herniated intravertebral discs, osteophytes, bone fragments, arachnoiditis, etc. The pain extends into the distribution of one or several adjacent nerve roots and is usually associated with other signs of nerve root involvement, such as sensory loss or deep tendon reflex abnormalities.

|Though central neuropathic pain is rarely seen in other conditions, it is the most common type of pain experienced by patients with spinal cord disease, especially patients with SCI. The pain is usually burning in quality and occurs mainly in the perineum and legs. Many patients with SCI rate this type of pain as their major disability. The mechanism by which central neuropathic pain is generated within the spinal cord (or brain) is unknown.[3]

Treatment
|Obviously the best treatment for any type of pain is removal of the cause. This is sometimes possible, i.e., stabilization of a fracture/dislocation, removal of a disk or spinal tumor, etc. However, in most instances, pain must be managed pharmacologically with analgesics, anticonvulsants, and antidepressants.[4]

|Nociceptive pain responds well to analgesic medication. Analgesics may act on the peripheral or central nervous system portions of the pain pathways. Peripherally acting analgesics produce their effect mainly by blocking the formation of the algesic substances, which depolarize the pain receptor. Aspirin, first used a century ago, was the first peripherally acting analgesic. During the past 30 years, and especially during the past 10 years, about 20 new peripherally acting analgesics have come to market. The peripherally acting analgesics are categorized as non-steroidal anti-inflammatory drugs (NSAIDs). Some examples of this group of drugs include ibuprofen, naproxen, piroxicam, and salindac. The newer drugs produce fewer side effects than aspirin but are much more expensive ($1 to $2 per tablet). A limitation of the peripherally acting analgesics is the "ceiling effect," e.g., 1,000 mg of aspirin produces all of the pain relief obtainable from aspirin; similarly 400 mg of ibuprofen produces all of the pain relief that can be obtained from ibuprofen. Because these drugs all work by the same mechanisms, combinations of peripherally acting analgesics cannot overcome the "ceiling effect," e.g., 1,000 mg of aspirin plus 400 mg of ibuprofen is no more effective than either drug administered alone.

|Centrally acting analgesics produce their effect by inhibiting pain transmission from the incoming peripheral nerve pain fiber to the dorsal horn neuron whose axon will carry the pain impulse to the brain or brain stem. They may produce this inhibition by direct action on synaptic sites within the dorsal horn or by activating descending inhibitory pathways originating in the brain stem, which terminate on synaptic sites in the dorsal horn. The centrally acting analgesics include the naturally occurring and synthetic opioids. Some commonly used opioids include morphine, butorphanol (Stadol), codeine, hydromorphone (Dilaudid), meperidine (Demerol), methadone (Dolophine), pentazocine (Talwin), propoxyphene (Darvon), etc.

|Because peripherally acting and centrally acting analgesics interfere with pain transmission at different sites and by different mechanisms, they may be used in combinations that produce more pain relief than is possible with either type of analgesic alone. Examples of such combinations are codeine/aspirin (Empirin Compound), oxycodone/aspirin (Percodan), propoxyphene/aspirin (Darvon Compound), etc.

|Acetaminophen is an analgesic used almost as long as aspirin. It has been difficult to classify regarding its mechanism of action though it is probably primarily peripheral. It is an excellent analgesic best known under the brand name of Tylenol. Combinations with centrally acting analgesics are widely used, e.g., with hydrocodone (Vicodin), with oxycodone (Percocet), etc.

|Tricyclic antidepressants, particularly amitriptyline (Elavil), are widely used in the management of chronic nociceptive pain. These drugs increase the amounts of synaptic serotonin and norepinephrine, both of which inhibit transmission within the central pain pathways. Norepinephrine is probably the more important of these inhibitory neurotransmitters because the selective serotonin reuptake inhibitors (SSRIs) do not seem useful in pain management.

|Peripheral neuropathic pain is thought to arise from ectopic generation of action potentials at the site of nerve injury, which then pass into and through central nervous system pain pathways. Perhaps other mechanisms are involved as well. Some anticonvulsants stabilize nerve cell membranes, which may explain their usefulness in the management of peripheral neuropathic pain, particularly if a lancinating quality is involved. Carbamazepine (Tegretol) seems to be the most effective anticonvulsant for pain management. Phenytoin (Dilantin) is less effective. Over the past several years, a number of publications have reported that gabapentin (Neurontin) is effective in the management of peripheral neuropathic pain, particularly that associated with diabetic neuropathy and post-herpetic neuralgia. Peripheral neuropathic pain also responds to treatment with centrally acting analgesics and tricyclic antidepressants.

|Unfortunately, the most common and most disabling type of pain associated with spinal cord disease, central neuropathic pain, is also the most resistant to treatment.[5] Because the mechanism by which the pain is generated is unknown, treatment is totally empirical. Peripherally acting analgesics are not useful. Opioids, tricyclic antidepressants, and anticonvulsants (carbamazepine, phenytoin, and gabapentin) have all been reported to be effective in some patients but not effective in others. Surgical ablation of pain pathways and stimulation of various central nervous system structures have generally not been helpful, with some exceptions. Acupuncture has been used with variable results.[6]

References

1. Fields HL. *Pain*. McGraw-Hill: New York, 1987.

2. Woolsey RM. Pain in spinal cord disorders. In: Young RR, Woolsey RM (Eds). *Diagnosis and Management of Disorders of the Spinal Cord*. WB Saunders: Philadelphia, 1995.

3. Christensen MD, Hulsebosch CE. Chronic central pain after spinal cord injury. *J Neurotrauma* 1997;14:517-537.

4. Balazy TE. Clinical management of chronic pain in spinal cord injury. *Clin J Pain* 1992;8:102-110.

5. Leijon G, Boivie J. Pharmacological treatment of central pain. In: Casey KL (Ed). *Pain and Central Nervous System Disease: The Central Pain Syndromes*. Raven Press: New York, 1991, pp. 257-266.

6. Ezzo J, et al. Is acupuncture effective for the treatment of chronic pain? A systemic review. *Pain* 2000;86(3):217-225.

Management of
LONG-BONE FRACTURES
in Patients With SCI

Douglas Garland, MD;
Leslie Shokes, MD

CHAPTER FIFTEEN ▰▰▰▰▰

Treatment principles for hip and long-bone fractures in spinal cord injury (SCI) have evolved over the years due to a better understanding of pathologic fractures and better internal fixation techniques. The potential exists for increased numbers of pathologic fractures, presently due to increased longevity and activity.

In 1962, Comarr[1] divided the treatment of long-bone fractures into four groups:

    I. Fractured upper extremity (UE) concomitant with cord injury
    II. Fractured lower extremity (LE) concomitant with cord injury
    III. Fractured UE after cord injury
    IV. Fractured LE after cord injury

He recommended that fracture management for injuries above the level of injury be treated as if the patient had no SCI. Treatment modalities for fractures below the level of injury were determined by the completeness of the neurologic lesion. Patients with incomplete injuries and functioning extremities required the same principles of fracture management as the general population. A splinting program was advised for most fractures and circular cast and operative management were discouraged secondary to complications. Because most patients with SCI did not ambulate, angular deformities and shortening of the LE were considered to be of no clinical consequences.

|The next advancement in fracture management occurred 10 years later.[2] Patients with SCI were divided into three groups:

    I. Fracture sustained in the same accident as the SCI.

    II. Fracture occurred in osteoporotic bone of patients with chronic SCI.

    III. Fracture in a chronic SCI caused by high energy.

Based on the results of their outcome, the following treatment recommendations were made:

Group 1: Treat long-bone fractures with open reduction and internal fixation (ORIF).

Group 2: When minimal specific treatment is needed, ORIF is usually contraindicated.

Group 3: Treat by methods that are least likely to disrupt the patient's lifestyle in a wheelchair.

Fractures in Acute SCI [3-5]

|Patients with acute cord injuries and concomitant long-bone fractures commonly have other associated injuries and demand complex medical and nursing care. Programs for skin, bowel, and bladder care, and eventually rehabilitation, are necessary. Therefore, the management of these acute fractures should facilitate nursing and medical care and rehabilitation without compounding the patient's disability. Fracture treatment should also produce a high rate of union, maintain length, prevent angular deformities, and maximize functional return.[6]

General

|Because high-energy accidents often cause multiple injuries, emergent stabilization of these organ systems is vital prior to treatment of the extremity fractures.[7, 8] Femur fractures are the most common long-bone injury followed by tibia fractures, humerus, radius, and ulna fractures. Recent data at specific LE fracture sites have shown improved outcome with operative stabilization regardless of the neurological status.

Femur

|Twenty-seven femoral shaft fractures were recently reviewed.[6] Fracture outcome was evaluated in the complete and incomplete groups as well as operative vs. non-operative fractures. One-third of the non-operative femurs displayed a tendency toward non-union. Angular and shortening deformities were also significantly higher compared to the operative group. Decubitus ulcers in the non-operative group were more severe and required a higher number of surgical procedures than those occurring in the operative group, resulting in additional bedrest.[9,10] Early operative stabilization of femoral shaft fractures was the preferred method of treatment regardless of the patient's neurologic status. Finally, non-operative fractures demonstrated a decreased healing potential that is in contradistinction to the general consensus.

Tibia

|The outcome of 34 tibia fractures in acute SCI was also the subject of a recent report. Fractures treated non-operatively healed at a prolonged rate with nearly 50% proceeding to delayed union or non-union. ORIF enhanced the rate and time to union. Except for type-III open injuries, fractures treated with early ORIF had the least orthopedic and medical complications. Routine ORIF of tibia fractures in both incomplete as well as complete SCI was advocated.[4] Patients with incomplete SCI routinely became ambulatory with orthopedic devices. Freedom from shortening and angular deformities facilitated this orthotic care.

Upper Extremity

|Fifty-three long-bone UE fractures were evaluated.[5] No significant difference between non-operative and operative treatment was detected with respect to time to union, rehabilitation, range of motion, or orthopedic complications when standard orthopedic fracture management principles were followed. The incidence of medical complications, such as deep venous thrombosis and decubitus ulcers, occurred more frequently in the non-operatively treated group. Early operative treatment is preferred for these fractures, unless closed treatment can be carried out predictably with a functional orthosis allowing the patient to participate in the rehabilitation process.

|The trend toward ORIF of all long-bone fractures in acute SCI has been evolving over decades. Initially, all fractures were treated non-operatively. Later, non-operative treatment was reserved for complete injuries with functionless extremities. Recent studies have demonstrated that non-operative treatment retards healing and leads to shortening and angular deformities. Presently, most LE fractures should undergo ORIF whether neurologically complete or incomplete. UE fracture care should follow general orthopedic principles with a tendency toward ORIF.

Fractures in Chronic SCI (Pathological Fractures)

|Fractures in patients with established SCI are usually caused by relatively minor injuries, although, major accidents may occur.[11] Patients with paraplegia have a higher incidence of fractures than patients with quadriplegia.[12] This difference results from the greater degree of function, mobility, and participation in various physical activities. The fracture rate is 10 times greater in individuals with complete lesions of the cord compared to those with incomplete lesions.[13] The overall incidence of pathologic fractures in patients with chronic SCI treated at SCI centers has been reported at 1.4% to 6%. This is probably a low estimate because many patients are treated locally and/or as outpatients and do not report to SCI centers. Many patients with trivial swelling in "painless" extremities may never seek medical attention.

|Patients with established SCI have numerous altered physiologic factors that affect the management of long-bone fractures. These patients have negative nitrogen and calcium balance as well as impaired skin sensitivity resulting in a propensity to develop decubitus ulcers, along with poor wound and fracture healing. They may have ongoing frequent urinary tract infections and bacteremia. Superficial and deep wound infections should be anticipated. Marked lower extremity spasticity may cause significant angular and rotary deformities, displacement of fracture fragments, as well as penetration of the fracture fragments through the skin. Significant spasticity may preclude use of non-operative management for shaft fractures. Casts may cause skin breakdown and splints may not provide adequate immobilization. On the other hand, osteoporosis may prevent adequate fixation.[4,14]

|Males with complete chronic SCI lose 33% of the bone mineral density (BMD) at the knee within a year of injury. Females with complete SCI lose 40% to 45% of their BMD within a year of their injury. Patients with known LE fracture have a 50% or greater loss of BMD at their knee. This 50% reduction of BMD at the knee seems to be the fracture threshold for this population. Females with SCI are at fracture risk at the knee soon after SCI. These populations should be counseled regarding osteoporosis and potential for fracture. Unexplained limb swelling, especially knee and ankle swelling, should cause them to seek medical attention.[5,14,15]

|At Rancho Los Amigos National Rehabilitation Center (RLANRC), a review of all patients with chronic SCI and a pathologic fracture from 1991 to 1995 was undertaken. There were 99 patients with fractures. The fracture location varied, but the overwhelming anatomic location was in the lower extremity. A breakdown of LE fractures revealed the supracondylar femur, followed closely by the proximal tibia, had the highest concentrations. All of the fractures united and, based upon this review, fracture management guidelines in this patient population were developed.

General

|Supracondylar fractures of the femur are the most commonly encountered, followed by proximal tibial and then tibial shaft fractures. The high incidence in these regions is consistent with the loss of bone mineral in these regions. The cause of the fracture was frequently a fall out of wheelchair on the osteoporotic part of the knee and torsion to the LE.

Hip

|Displaced femoral neck fractures are uncommon, but pose a difficult management dilemma. If left untreated, the femur may migrate proximally, unbalancing the pelvis and causing pressure sores.[16] Displaced femoral neck fractures result in non-union, even when reduced and pinned, because fixation failure occurs. Prosthetic replacement may be prudent, although dislocation after surgery may occur as well as late subluxation and dislocation. Acetabular erosion may result from osteoporotic bone. Outcomes of cementing of the prosthesis vs. bony ingrowth have not been determined.

|Intertrochanteric fractures with pin and side plate may result in failure of fixation due to the osteoporosis. Non-operative management is associated with varus deformity of the hip, which is often acceptable. The new intramedullary hip fixation devices offer an improved fixation technique that is currently the preferred operative method if surgery is deemed necessary.[17]

Femoral Shaft

|Femoral shaft fractures may be very difficult to manage non-operatively, especially in patients with spasticity. Non-unions are commonplace in displaced fractures, as has been established in the acute SCI population. Casts and splints are frequently inadequate. External fixation, although effective, is not without its own set of complications, such as pin infection fixation failure through osteoporotic bone and stress fracture through the pin site at a later date. Immobilization by external fixation may interfere with patient positioning and predispose to trophic ulcers.[18] The treatment of choice for displaced femoral fractures or non-displaced fracture, which lose reduction during non-operative methods, is interlocking, intramedullary rodding. Locking is necessary because the femoral canals are wide and rotational deformities as well as non-union cannot be prevented with standard nails.

Distal Femur/Proximal Tibia

|These minimally or non-displaced fractures are the most commonly encountered fractures in this patient population. Well-padded splints or a knee immobilizer are the best methods of treatment.[19] They provide adequate immobilization along with a low incidence of skin breakdown. Frequent inspection of the skin is required. Pillow splints have been widely used in the past, but are bulky and make mobilization difficult. Long leg casts are not recommended, but are occasionally used when these other non-operative methods fail. Surgery for displaced fractures may be necessary.[20] Retrograde intramedullary nails through the knee is advantageous.

Tibial Shaft

|Management of tibial shaft fractures can be treated non-operatively if minimally or non-displaced. Displaced fractures require interlocking intramedullary fixation.

Ankle

|Ankle fractures are usually low-energy fracture patterns. These fractures can be treated with a padded posterior splint or cam walker. Healing may be either bony or fibrous union without complications. Varus-valgus angular deformities are unacceptable because malleolar pressure sores may ensue.

Foot

|Metatarsal base and toe fractures are usually non-displaced and unite with a soft splint without consequence. Splinting in equinus position may lead to a fixed deformity.

Upper Extremity

|Preservation of UE function is especially important in these patients. Management of pathologic fractures that only occur in the aged SCI population and on occasional patients with quadriparesis should follow general orthopedic principles with an emphasis on preserving function. Bone mineral loss is not significant and fixation devices are not prone to failure.

Conclusion

|A high index of suspicion of an extremity fracture is necessary in the assessment of patients who are paralyzed who develop a swollen extremity. A careful history of any trauma, however minor, should be carefully sought in patients with SCI, spina bifida, and end-stage multiple sclerosis. Late-onset swelling may be the only sign to diagnosis. Other general signs, such as an increase in spasticity or sweating or dysreflexia, should also alert the clinician to the possibility of an occult fracture.

|Management of extremity fractures in patients with pathologic fractures varies depending on the location. Hip fractures continue to be a difficult management problem due to the poor fixation obtained in the osteoporotic bone with current fixation devices. Some intertrochanteric, subtrochanteric, and femoral fractures should be managed with interlocking, intramedullary nails, if technically possible. Distal femoral and proximal tibial fractures can be treated with well-padded splints. Most displaced tibial shaft fractures require an interlocking, intramedullary nail. Distal tibia, ankle, and foot fractures respond to splinting. UE fracture management should follow general orthopedic principles.

Editor's Note

|This chapter was written by a world authority in spinal cord surgeries. We would like to caution the enthusiastic resident not to schedule fractures of the LE for ORIF without consultation with a senior expert. In our experience, a small percentage of closed LE fractures needed an intervention, ORIF, or external fixation, particularly in complete injuries. These procedures are not free from complications, caution against circular casts, skin or skeletal traction. In our center, we developed a custom-made splint (Long Beach Splint) made of canvas lined with sheepskin and supported by wooden ribs to prevent folding. It permits skin inspections and radiography without removing it.

|In our center, non-invasive electromagnetic stimulation has helped union in many cases. In any insensate limb, the skin must always be inspected for breakdown, callus formation, and fracture healing. We use EBI machine for home use and Diapulse in hospitals or nursing home settings.

References

1. Comarr A, Hutchinson R, Bors E. Extremity fracture of patients with spinal cord injuries. *Am J Surg* 1962;103:732.

2. McMaster W, Stauffer ES. The management of long bone fracture in the spinal cord injured patient. *Clin Orthop* 1975;112:44.

3. Garland D, Reiser T, Singer D. Treatment of femoral shaft fractures associated with acute spinal cord injuries. *Clin Orthop* 1985;197:191.

4. Garland D, Saucedo T, Reiser T. The management of tibial fractures in acute spinal cord injury patients. *Clin Orthop* 1986;213:237.

5. Garland D, Jones R, Kunkle R. Upper extremity fractures in the acute spinal cord injury patients. *Clinic Orthop* 1988;233:110.

6. Eichenholtz S. Management of long-bone fractures in paraplegic patients. *J Bone Joint Surg* 1963;45A:299.7.

7. Sobel M, Lyden J. Long bone fracture in a spinal cord injured patient. *J Trauma* 1991;31:1440.

8. Levine A, Krebs M, Santos-Mendoza N. External fixation in quadriplegia. *Clin Orthop* 1984;184:169.

9. Baird R, Kreitenberg A. Treatment of femoral shaft fractures in the spinal cord injury patient using the Wagner leg lengthening device. *Paraplegia* 1984;22:366.

10. Freehafer A, Hazel C, Becker C. Lower extremity fractures in patients with spinal cord injury. *Paraplegia* 1951;19:367.

11. Keating JF, Ken M, Delorgy M. Minimal trauma causing fractures in patients with spinal cord injury. *Disability and Rehabilitation* 1992;14:108.

12. Ragnarsson K, Sell GH. Lower extremity fractures after spinal cord injury: a retrospective study. *Arch Phys Med Rehab* 1981;62:418.

13. Ingram RR, Suman RK, Freeman MA. Lower limb fractures in the chronic spinal cord injury patient. *Paraplegia* 1989;27:133.

14. Garland D, Stewart C, Adkins R, et al. Osteoporosis after spinal cord injury. *J Orthop Research* 1992;10:371.

15. Garland D, Maric Z, Adkins R, Stewart C. Bone mineral density about the knee in spinal cord injured patients with pathological fractures. *Contemp Orthop* 1993;26:375.

16. Garland D. Clinical observations on fractures and heterotopic ossification in the spinal cord and traumatic brain injured population. *Clin Orthop* 1988;233:86.

17. Rimoldi RC, Capen DA. Thigh compartment syndrome secondary to intertrochanteric hip fracture in a quadriplegic patient. *Paraplegia* 1992;30:376.

18. Baird R, Kreitenberg A, Eltorai I. External fixation of femoral shaft fractures in spinal cord injury patients. *Paraplegia* 1986;24:183.

19. El Ghatit A, Lamid S, Flathy T. Posterior splint for leg fractures in spinal cord injured patients. *Am J Phys Med* 1981;60:239.

20. Freehafer A, Mast W. Lower extremity fractures in patients with spinal cord injury. *J Bone Joint Surg* 1965;47A:683.

DISLOCATIONS
Ibrahim M. Eltorai, MD

in the Lower Extremities

CHAPTER SIXTEEN ▰▰▰▰▰▰▰▰

|The most common dislocation in patients with spinal cord injury (SCI) is the hip dislocation. Hip dislocations in the these patients are divided into three groups.

I. Septic hip dislocation: This is the most common and is caused by pyarthrosis secondary to pressure ulcer extension into the joint. Due to sepsis into the joint, the capsule and ligaments are destroyed, the bone is infected and may be destroyed, including the femoral head and the acetabulum. Infection usually aggravates spasticity in upper motor neuron lesions, especially hip flexors and adductors, which initiate the dislocation, usually a dorsal dislocation and frequently into the ulcer itself. Surgical intervention on decubiti, especially with debridement of soft tissues around the hip, including the muscle and partial ostectomies, may predispose to the dislocation. This is predominant in children with SCI.[1]

II. Non-septic hip dislocation: The exact etiology is not clear, however, the following factors contribute to the occurrence of the dislocation:

    A. Spasticity: Persistent adductor and flexor spasticity stretch the capsule of the joint and possibly erode the posterior acetabular rim.

    B. Scoliosis and pelvic obliquity may be a contributing factor.

    C. Possibly recurrent minor trauma such as falls.

    D. Possibly prolonged standing in a frame.

    E. Advanced degrees of muscle wasting are questionable factors.

    F. Pre-existing acetabular anomalies are hard to document.[2]

    G. Pathological femoral neck fracture due to osteoporosis.

III. Traumatic dislocation is rare and is similar to hip dislocation in individuals without paralysis. Recurrent dislocation has been reported, but no major trauma was causative.[3]

Types of Dislocation

I. Simple dislocations:

    A. Posterior is the most common.

    B. Anterior is less common.

    C. Central is very rare, and is due to major trauma caused by accidents.

II. Fracture dislocations: Dislocations associated with fractures of any of the constituents of the hip or below it.

Symptoms

|Except in the traumatic cases, there may be no symptoms. Symptoms usually are: pain, discomfort, swelling, increasing spasticity, diminution of the sitting tolerance and/or sitting balance, and increasing frequency and pattern of pressure sores, which develop mostly on the contralateral side. Autonomic dysreflexia may be the first manifestation and may be persistent until the dislocation is treated. In one case, cardiac arrhythmia was the first manifestation. Transferring to the wheelchair may be difficult. In case of septic arthritis due to pressure ulcers, for example, the dislocation may be evident by inspection and/or palpation of the ulcer. X-rays are diagnostic of any type of dislocation.

Treatment

    I. Preventive:

        A. Septic hips should be prevented by avoiding pressure sores, and if they develop on the hip they should be treated energetically by surgery or otherwise.

        B. Non-septic hip subluxation can be prevented by:

            i. Treatment of spasticity pharmacologically, including baclofen pump if needed.

            ii. The use of nerve blocks or neurosurgical intervention.

            iii. Tendon release, especially hip flexor and adductor groups.

            iv. Physical therapy: Passive stretching, hydrotherapy, and knee spreading.

            v. Patients who use a standing frame over long periods of time should be observed not only for spasticity, but also periodic X-rays of the pelvis should be taken. If the acetabulum is shallow or its rim eroded, they should discontinue standing.

II. Therapeutics:

    A. Non-septic dislocation: In symptomatic patients, treatment is by attempting closed reduction after tendon release and relief of spasticity (See chapter 13 on spasticity).[4] If it recurs, shelving of the acetabulum plus tenotomies may be tried as well as reconstruction of the ligamentum teres using carbon fiber. This is especially applicable in ambulatory patients (incomplete injuries). In absence of symptoms, especially in complete injuries, no treatment is needed, only follow-up.

    B. Radical procedure: In ambulatory patients, Girdlestone operation with or without arthroplasty is indicated in painful joint dislocation. The latter is liable to fail due to osteoporosis and infection. In septic cases, upper femorectomy (Girdlestone procedure) will have to be done, filling or packing the resulting cavity by a muscle, most commonly the vastus externus and/or gluteus maximus.[5]

|Fracture dislocations will require open reduction and internal fixation in non-septic cases. In one case, the fracture dislocation occurred through a pressure sore for which upper femorectomy was done.

|Other dislocations of the lower extremities are very rare and are associated with fractures due to severe trauma and usually open injuries. These are managed by aggressive orthopedic procedures and may end by amputation.

Conclusion

|Dislocations of the lower extremities in patients with SCI are most common in the hip. This is mostly due to extension of infection from pressure ulcers around the joint with secondary destruction of joint capsule or infection of the upper femoral end. The non-septic group is mostly due to the patient's uncontrolled spasticity, skeletal deformities, and possibly repeated trauma and weight bearing. The third type is due to major trauma. In septic cases, Girdlestone procedure is recommended. In non-septic cases, if they are symptomatic, the same procedure is usually needed. Hip replacement is of doubtful value in patients with SCI.

References

1. Evans GRD, Lewis Jr VL, Manson PN, et al. Hip joint complication with pressure sore: The refractory wound and the role of Girdlestone arthroplasty. *Plastic Reconstr Surg* 1993;912:288-294.

2. Baird RA, DeBenedetti MJ, Eltorai I. Nonseptic hip instability in the chronic spinal cord injury patient. *Paraplegia* 1986:24(5):293-300.

3. Rockwood Jr CA, Green DP. Dislocations and fracture dislocations of the hip. *Rockwood and Green's Fractures in Adults,* Third Edition, Vol 2. JB Lippincott Co.: Philadelphia, 1991; pp. 1574-1625.

4. Eltorai IM, Montroy R. Muscle release in the management of spasticity in spinal cord injury. *Paraplegia* 1990:28:433-440.

5. Eltorai IM. Girdlestone procedure in spinal cord injury. *J Amer Paraplegia Society* 1983;6:85-86.

OSTEOMYELITIS
Due to Pressure Ulcers

CHAPTER SEVENTEEN ▬▬▬▬▬▬▬ | *Ibrahim M. Eltorai, MD*

|Bone infections are currently classified by Waldvogel et al as follows:[1,2]

I. Hematogenous osteomyelitis is divided to acute and chronic according to the sequence of the disease. This is usually a disease of childhood and rare in adults. This is not applicable to pressure ulcers.

II. Osteomyelitis secondary to a contiguous focus of infection (pressure ulcers or other adjacent soft-tissue infections).[3-5] It also develops after trauma or surgical intervention. This class is subdivided into:

A. Osteomyelitis with vascular insufficiency. The majority of patients are diabetic. The onset is usually after infections of the feet where perfusion is inadequate and blunting of the local tissue response has occurred. The infection may start in a trophic pressure ulcer or after trauma or surgery. In a population with spinal cord injury (SCI), studies showed that 20% have vascular compromise of some degree. (See chapter 12 on acute arterial occlusion.)

B. Osteomyelitis without vascular compromise. This is the type that complicates pressure ulcers. There is another classification (Cierny & Mader) that is non-applicable to pressure ulcer cases.[6, 7]

|Our classification with pressure ulcers is as follows:

i. Periostitis: usually seen with ulcers on the malleoli, on the shin, and the olecranon.

ii. Osteoperiostitis: this is a further stage of the above grade.

iii. Osteomyelitis: seen in the trochanter, ischia, and calcaneous bones, coccyx and/or sacrum, and metatarsals.

|The organisms most commonly encountered are coagulase-positive and negative Staphylococcus aureus, streptococcus species, Gram-negative bacilli, and occasionally anaerobes, especially in the ischial bones due to fecal contamination.[8] However, mixed infections are common. The sites involved are the ischia, coccyx, sacrum, trochanter, heel, malleoli, toe, olecranon, and the spine, in descending order.

Clinical Presentation

|The onset may be acute with abscess formation and signs of septicemia or even septic shock. Most commonly, the presentation is subacute or chronic. Low-grade fever and signs of local infection are usually evident. In the chronic form, some degree of intermittent pyrexia—especially in the evenings, loss of appetite, anemia, and increasing spasms are often present. Local examination may show exposed necrotic bone, sequestra, pyogenic loculi, and sinus formation. The presentation may be worse with health compromise, e.g., diabetes mellitus, renal failure, malnutrition, immunosupression, chronic hypoxia, especially with tobacco abuse, drug abuse, and depression.

Diagnosis is based on:

I. Clinical findings.

II. Laboratory findings: Leucocytosis with shift to the left, unexplained anemia, high sedimentation rate, wound and bone biopsy for culture, and histopathology are often positive. In febrile patients, blood cultures are repeatedly taken, but are not always positive.

III. X-rays usually show lytic areas in particular bones, bone thickening, periosteal reaction, and spread to a neighboring joint.[9] A sinogram is indicated with sinus formation.

IV. Computed tomography shows increased marrow density and may help identify areas of necrotic bone as well as soft-tissue infection.[10,11]

V. In difficult cases, MRI helps differentiate between bone and soft-tissue infection.

VI. Radionuclide testing will show increased blood flow and reactive bone formation. Usually technicium scan (99TE) is followed by gallium scan. Indium-labeled leucocytes may show the site of bone infection. Gallium and indium attach to transferrin that leaks from blood in inflamed areas. In our experience, the radionuclides are non-conclusive: they do not show bone detail well because increased uptake occurs in soft-tissue infection. We depend mostly on radiography and bone biopsy. Indium leucocyte scan is positive in 40% of cases of acute osteomyelitis and 60% of cases of septic arthritis.[12] In chronic osteomyelitis, it is usually negative.

|As an emergency, patients usually present a picture of sepsis and abscess formation; sometimes with spread into a neighboring joint, especially the hip with septic arthritis. We have encountered a few cases with paravertebral suppuration due to osteomyelitis of the spine secondary to sacral or lumbar pressure ulcers. One case led to a pneumocephalus.

Management

Antibiotic therapy: This should be initiated when the bone culture and sensitivity are obtained. If the patient is ill, then empiric, broad-spectrum antibiotics may be started and modified if necessary after sensitivities are obtained. Adequate drainage is necessary and may be accompanied by debridement. The antibiotics have to be continued intravenously for 4 to 6 weeks.[13] If there is not an easy access, an alternative long-term access needs to be adopted (See chapter 11 on venous access). Oral therapy using quinolones may be used for Gram-negative organisms, but not against strep species, enterocci, and staph species. Oral antibiotic therapy should be preceded by 2 weeks of intravenous therapy (See the antibiotic therapy chapter in *Emergencies of Pressure Ulcers*).

|When infection is under control, appropriate surgical repair of the wound is mandatory. After ostectomy, filling the dead space with different kinds of flaps is necessary.[14] Antibacterial impregnated acrylic beads have rarely been used.[15] To be sure that all infected bone is removed, tetracycline tagging is recommended. The patient is given tetracycline, 250 mg orally every 6 hours for 4 to 5 days before surgery. (After bone removal, Wood's lamp is used to see fluorescence of the healthy bone after debridement.) If the case is not treated, then the patient is liable to exacerbations and extension into the joint space. Bone marrow suppression with anemia, amyloid disease, and malignancy may complicate chronic cases.

|Hyperbaric oxygen therapy may be used as an adjunctive therapy.[16-22] This increases oxygen tension in the infected tissue, including the bone. This is necessary for the polymorphonuclear cells' killing function, for bacteriostasis of anaerobes, for angiogenesis, and fibroblast cellular activity for wound healing. It may help in patients with vascular insufficiency.

Surgical procedures in special sites: Osteomyelitis of the hip requires upper femorectomy (Girdlestone procedure).[23-24] No hip replacements are done in a septic field, especially in patients with complete SCI.

Amputations are rarely indicated for:

    I. Osteomyelitis of the toe.

    II. Ischemic extremities, especially in diabetes when revascularization is not possible.

    III. Contracted deformed extremity when repair is not possible.

    IV. Septic ankle or knee when conservative measures failed.

    V. Fracture at the site of osteomyelitis.

    VI. Marjolin's ulcer.

|Amputation should never be done for osteomyelitis of the upper extremity. Preservation of the limb with a wound or sinus is more acceptable than amputation.

References

1. Waldvogel FA, Medoff C, Swartz MN. Osteomyelitis: a review of clinical features, therapeutic considerations, and unusual aspects. *N Engl J Med* 1970;282:198-206, 316-322.

2. Waldvogel FA, Vasey H. Osteomyelitis: the past decade. *N Engl J Med* 1980;303: 360-370.

3. Lewis Jr. VL, Bailey MH, Pulawski G, et al. The diagnosis of osteomyelitis in patients with pressure sores. *Plastic and Recon Surg* 1988;81(2):229-232.

4. Sugarman B, Hawes S, Musher DM, et al. Osteomyelitis beneath pressure sores. *Arch Int Med* 1983;143:683-688.

5. Thornhill-Joynes M, Gonzales F, Stewart CA, et al. Osteomyelitis associated with pressure ulcers. *Arch PM&R* 1986:67.

6. Cierny G, Mader JT. Adult chronic osteomyelitis. *Orthopedics* 1984;7:1557-1564.

7. Cierny G, Mader JT, Pennick H. A clinical staging system of adult osteomyelitis. *Contemp Ortho* 1985;10:17-37.

8. Mandell GL, Bennett JE, Dolin R. *Principles and practice of infectious diseases* 1995;Churchill Livingstone: pp.1039-1050.

9. Hendrix RW, Calenoff L, Ledermann RB, Neiman HL. Radiology of pressure sores. *Radiology* 1981;138:351.

10. Firooznai H, Rafii M, Golimbu C, et al. Computerized tomography of pelvic osteomyelitis, pressure sores, pelvic abscess in spinal cord injury patients. *Arch Phys Med Rehab* 1982;63:545-548.

11. Seltzer SE. Value of computed tomography in planning medical and surgical treatment of chronic osteomyelitis. *J Comput Assist Tomogr* 1984;8(3):482-487.

12. Propst-Proctor SL, Dillingham MF, Mcdougall IR, Goodwin D. The white blood scan in orthopedics. *Clin Ortho* 1982;168:157-165.

13. Van Rens JG, Kayser FH. Local antibiotic treatment in osteomyelitis and soft tissue infections. Proceedings of a symposium, Oct 25, 1980: *Excerpta Medica*, 1981: Amsterdam-Oxford-Princeton.

14. Ruttle PE, Kelly PJ, Arnold PG, et al. Chronic osteomyelitis treated with muscle flap. *Orthop Clin North Amer* 1984;15(3):451-458.

15. Hedstrom S, Lidgren L, Torham C, Onnerfalt R. Antibiotic containing bone cement beads in the treatment of deep muscle and skeletal infections. *Acta Orthop Scand* 51:863-869.

16. Campagnolo DI, Barlett JA, Keller SE, et al. Impaired phagocytosis of staphylococcugaureus in complete tetraplegia. *Phys Med & Rehab* 1997;76(4):276-280.

17. Eltorai I, Hart GB, Strauss MB. Osteomyelitis in the spinal cord injured. A review and preliminary report on the use of hyperbaric oxygen therapy. *Paraplegia* 1984;22:17-24.

18. Mader JT, Adams KR, Sutton TE. Infectious diseases:pathophysiology and mechanisms of hyperbaric oxygen. *J Hyperbaric Medicine* 1987;2:133-140.

19. Morrey, BF, Dunn Jm, Heimbach RD, et al. Hyperbaric oxygen and chronic osteomyelitis. *Clinical Ortho* 1979;144:121-127.

20. Mader JT. Bacterial. *Osteomyelitis, hyperbaric oxygen therapy: Critical review.* Undersea & Medical Soc. Inc.; Bethesda, MD 1991: 75-94.

21. Calhoun JH, Cobos JA, Mader JT. Does hyperbaric oxygen have a place in the treatment of osteomyelitis? *Ortho Clin N Amer* 1991;22(3):467-471.

22. Britt M, Calhoun J, Mader JT, Mader JP. The use of hyperbaric oxygen in the treatment of osteomyelitis. In: *Hyperbaric Medicine Practice*. Kindwal (Ed). Best Publishing Company: Flagstaff, AZ,1994; pp. 420-427.

23. Eltorai IM. Girdlestone procedure in spinal cord injury. *J Amer Paraplegia Soc* 1983;6(4):85-86.

24. Evans GRD, Lewis VL, Manson PN, Loomis M, Vander CA. Hip joint communication with pressure sore. The refractory wound and the role of Girdlestone arthroplasty. *Plast Reconstruct Surg* 1993;91(2):288-294.

DECUBITUS ULCER
Ibrahim M. Eltorai, MD; Rodney M. Wishnow, MD

Emergencies in Patients With SCI

CHAPTER EIGHTEEN ■■■■■■■■■■■■■■■■■■

Decubitus ulcers, or pressure sores, may sound simple but they can cause serious complications, or even a deadly outcome. The purpose of this chapter is to guide the caretakers of patients with spinal cord injury (SCI) through emergency situations due to pressure sores.

In a period of 18 years, 2,881 patients were admitted to the SCI Center at the Long Beach Department of VAMC with pressure sores as their main diagnosis. An almost equal number of patients were admitted with pressure sores as a secondary diagnosis. Approximately 10% had active infection with systemic manifestations. It is important to stress the fact that systemic infection in SCI can be very serious, especially in patients with poor nutrition, anemia, renal disease, liver disease, cardiovascular disease, chronic obstructive pulmonary disease, and diabetes mellitus. The source of systemic bacterial infection may be the pressure sore itself, or may be due to local complications, such as cellulitis, lymphangitis, septic thrombophlebitis, bursitis, osteomyelitis, and septic arthritis. Bacterial spread may follow trauma, surgical debridement, surgical excision, and rough handling.[1] Over time, it may also spread by its own advancement through neighboring tissue or blood vessel invasion, especially in a compromised patient.[2-3]

Infection Complications as Emergencies
Bloodstream infections: Spread of infection into the bloodstream is one of the most emergent complications of pressure sores. The clinical spectrum of blood infections can be divided into three major categories: bacteremias, septicemias, and septic shock. Sepsis generally is manifested by elevated temperature, tachycardia, tachypnea, leucocytosis, and the presence of immature bands in the peripheral blood.

I. Bacteremia is simply the presence of bacteria in the blood, as demonstrated by a positive blood culture.[4] A patient with bacteremia may or may not have symptoms and may have only a low-grade fever for which a blood culture was initially drawn. The duration and pattern of bacteremia may give a clue as to its source.

Transient bacteremia (lasting perhaps only a matter of minutes) occurs after instrumentation, dental extraction, or debridement of a pressure sore. It may occur with simple tooth-brushing or bowel care. In sustained bacteremia, blood cultures may be positive over several hours or days. This is suggestive of intravascular infection (endocarditis, phlebitis, or infected intravascular catheter, vascular graft). Intermittent bacteremia often occurs with genitourinary or biliary obstruction or episodic manipulation of an infected area. However, it may also be seen with the same conditions that cause sustained bacteremias. Chills and fever may occur for over an hour during which time the immune system may clear the blood of bacteria. The blood culture at the time of fever may be negative but it might have been positive for a half-hour to an hour before the spike and chill. The important issue is that intermittent bacteremias may not be identified by a single blood culture; blood cultures may need to be repeated 3, 6, or 8 times in order to detect bacteremia.[5-7]

II. Septicemia is a bacteremia along with clinical manifestations of severe infection, such as chills, fever, malaise, toxicity, and hypotension.

III. In septic shock, the patient's blood pressure is decreased by one-third of its previous level with decreased urinary output, decreased mentation, cool extremities, hypoxemia, and elevated lactate level.

|Septic shock is often described as occurring in two phases:

A. Early phase: Body temperature may be elevated or normal. There may be chills, a minor or slight decrease in blood pressure, tachycardia, rarely bradycardia, warm skin due to release of vasodilators, increased cardiac output and central venous pressure, and an altered mental status. This is the stage where the case should be energetically treated. This is also called the hyperdynamic or warm shock of sepsis.

B. Later phase (cold or hypodynamic shock): There is diminished sensorium, confusion and/or agitation, the skin is cold and clammy due to vasoconstriction and decreased central pressure, and urinary output is diminished. Decreased cardiac output and central venous pressure lead to severe hypotension and hypoxia. Adult respiratory distress syndrome may develop, and oliguria may progress to acute tubular necrosis. Hypoxia leads to metabolic (lactic) acidosis. The pathophysiology of sepsis is not simple, especially with Gram-negative organisms.

|The virulence of the Gram negatives is determined by lipopolysaccharide (LPS). This factor triggers humoral enzymatic mechanisms involving the complement, clotting, fibrinolytic, and kinin pathways. Fever and inflammation are mediated by cytokines that are released in response to LPS. Tumor Necrotizing Factors (TNF-α, interferon-y, interleukin-l [IL-l]) are produced within minutes or hours of contact between LPS and defense cells (monocytes or macrophages). IL-l and TNF-α are potent pyrogens. IL-6 is a mild pyrogen, IL-8 is chemotactic activating the neutrophils. IL-10 acts on the macrophages to down regulate TNF-α. TNF-α with other cytokines induces nitric oxide synthesase. Nitric oxide is a potent vasodilator that causes hypotension. In septicemias, cytokines play a major role in disseminated intravascular coagulopathy. For details please see reference.[8-10] In patients with SCI, natural and adaptive immune responses are decreased in the initial injury. Natural killer cell functions are also decreased. T-cell function and/or activities are decreased, but they improved through physical rehabilitation therapy.

|A substantial portion of the blood volume may be pooled in the venous capacitance bed, producing a relative hypovolemia. The "effective circulating blood volume" is thus decreased, leading to an increase in the release of catecholamines and an increase in the sympathetic tone and peripheral resistance. The shock is more profound in patients with dehydration, anemia, or cardiovascular disease. Complications may develop, especially hypotension, hemorrhages, leukopenia, thrombocytopenia, organ failure viz. cyanosis, acidosis, oliguria, anuria, jaundice, and congestive heart failure. These are to be expected in debilitated patients and are of grave significance. Disseminated intravascular coagulopathy indicates a bad prognosis. Bacteremias and septicemias are of particular concern to patients with SCI because of their:

    I. Abnormal neuroaxis
    II. Autonomic system hypersensitivity
    III. Altered hemodynamic system
    IV. Impaired respiratory capacity in patients with quadriplegia
    V. Tendency to anemia, hypoproteinemia, and possible hypovolemia
    VI. Risk for having more than one source for the bacteremia

|Several recent studies have shown the danger of bacteremia from pressure sores.[1-5] A study of 102 patients with bacteremia and pressure sores revealed the ulcers to be the possible source of bacteremia in 49% of the episodes; another site of infection was documented in 86% of the patients. The sacrum was the most common site of the associated pressure sore (52%), with the ischium (29%), heels (13%), and trochanter (12%) following behind. Multiplicity of the sores was encountered in 61% of the cases.

|The specific microorganism(s) causing bacteremia depends largely on the source of the primary infection. Bacteremias secondary to pressure sores are often due to Gram-negative bacilli, such as *Proteus mirabilis* or *Escherichia coli*, with *Staphylococcus aureus* and *Enterococcus* accounting for only about 10% to 20% and 5%, respectively.[2] This is possibly due to the fact that pressure sores are most commonly infected with *Proteus*, *E. coli*, and Gram-positive cocci. *Bacteroides* bacteremia is generally secondary to a pressure sore or gastrointestinal source. It may account for 12% to 50% of the pressure sore-associated bacteremias.[1,2] Ischial pressure ulcers complicated by Fournier's gangrene are common sources of *Bacteroides* infection. Fungemias, especially candidemia, are more commonly associated with infected lines or foreign bodies than with pressure sores. They may be due to pressure sores in patients who are colonized with *Candida* due to prolonged, broad-spectrum antibacterial therapy.

Other infectious complications: Some of the following infectious complications of pressure sores are themselves not emergencies. However, they require prompt treatment because they may rapidly spread locally or systemically (through the bloodstream). In other words, these urgencies may become emergencies if not brought under control.

I. Cellulitis or inflammation/infection of the skin and subcutaneous tissue. This is usually caused by *Streptococcus* or *Staphylococcus*; sometimes by *Proteus* or *Serratia*.

II. Lymphangitis, or spread of infection through the routes of lymph drainage, centrally towards lymph nodes. This pattern of spread may rapidly lead to blood-borne infection.

III. Fournier's gangrene, with progressive tissue necrosis, often involves anaerobic bacteria or mixed infections. It is a surgical as well as medical emergency.

IV. Septic bursitis, septic arthritis, and osteomyelitis generally result from direct extension of the pressure sore, although they may also occur as a result of seeding from the bloodstream. In our studies, osteomyelitis was found in 5% of patients.[5,11] The most common sites in descending order are: hips, ischia, sacrum, and calcanea.

Non-infectious emergencies:

I. Hemorrhage is rarely noted spontaneously but may occur after debridement. Hemorrhage is especially seen in patients who are anticoagulated pharmacologically (receiving warfarin, aspirin, or non-steroidal anti-inflammatory drug), congenitally (due to hemophilia, thrombocytopenia, von Willebrand's disease) or as a result of their underlying condition (uremic patients or patients receiving hemodialysis). The treatment is to ligate a visible bleeder or pack the wound with Gelfoam-Thrombin. If the problem persists, take the patient to the operating room for adequate hemostasis by the Bovi or laser beam. Transfusion may be needed. Fresh frozen plasma, cryoprecipitate, or Factor VIII may be indicated for coagulopathy.

II. Visceral involvement can represent, in a dramatic way, the potential complications of pressure sores. Extension of a pressure sore to involve the urethra may lead to a urinary fistula. This occurs particularly after total ischiectomy with the development of urethral diverticula. Emergency care is needed through the use of proper antibiotics and indwelling catheterization. In a few cases, suprapubic cystostomy and bladder neck ligation may be required. Fourteen such cases have been encountered with 10 being reported by the senior author.[12]

|The rectum may be involved, with perirectal infections, supralevator infection, rectal fistulae, and bacteremia. Incision and drainage with or without colostomy as a temporary or permanent measure may be required.

III. Autonomic dysreflexia may be triggered by pressure sores, especially during surgery, debridement, or even dressing change.[13] The appropriate treatment should be performed after ruling out other potential causes (i.e., bladder obstruction or infection, and rectal impaction). When relieving the cause is inadequate or impossible, medications may be required. Our course of treatment is a 10-mg nifedipine capsule, to be punctured and swallowed with close monitoring. (See chapter 1 on autonomic dysreflexia.)

Rare complications encountered:

I. Sacral ulcer eroding the dura, leading to fatal septic meningitis.

II. Sacral ulcer with extension into the pelvis, leading to pelvic cellulitis, septicemia, and death.

III. Sacral ulcer with extension paravertebrally up to the neck, necessitating multiple incisions.

IV. Sacral ulcer with extension of the infection into the pelvis and retroperitoneal space and also to the paravertebral planes. Treatment involved drainage in multiple procedures, antibiotics, colostomy, and hyperbaric oxygen therapy (HBO) for anaerobic infections.

V. Six cases of Fournier's gangrene (necrotizing perineal fasciitis) were treated by debridement, antibiotics, and HBO. One patient required colostomy. Fortunately, none of our patients suffered a fatal outcome. However, it should be remembered that the mortality of this serious infection is generally 25% to 50%.

VI. Lumbar ulcer eroding the dura with air suction leading to a pneumocephalus; patient survived surgical repair.

Assessment and Diagnosis

|Bacteremia must be considered when a patient with SCI develops a shaking chill followed by a rapid rise in temperature. The source of the infection may be the decubitus only, or it may be an associated urinary infection, pulmonary infection, or other source. Assessment begins with a detailed history and physical examination. A careful examination is essential because there may be more than one focus of infection. Do not be satisfied simply by finding a decubitus ulcer; other sources should always be ruled out.

|In a septic patient, routine blood work (complete blood count with differential count, blood chemistries) and urinalysis can reveal the extent of infection, as well as identify other underlying illnesses (dehydration, electrolyte abnormalities, anemia, liver disease, renal disease, or infection, etc.). These concurrent problems may have an impact upon the treatment course, antibiotic selection, and dosage.

|Wound cultures should be obtained. Wound swabs are the least valuable because they may simply represent colonizing bacteria that are likely to be present in ulcerated skin. Cultures of tissue or undrained pus are the most valuable source of culture material, and can usually be submitted for both aerobic and anaerobic evaluation. Tissue bacterial count is time-consuming and expensive.[14]

|Two or three sets of aerobic and anaerobic blood cultures should be drawn at least 30 minutes apart. Any other source that is likely to be infected (i.e., urine, sputum) should also be submitted for culture.

|X-rays of the ulcer site are appropriate to rule out bone and/or joint infection. However, early bone disease may not be identified by these studies. Nuclear medicine scans are frequently used to evaluate the possibility of osteomyelitis; yet, they are often non-specific and identify inflammation rather than infection. Tomography or CT scans are useful for detecting bone or joint infections. Where available, MRI is proving to be one of the most sensitive and specific tests for early detection of osteomyelitis and soft-tissue infections. (See chapter 17 on osteomyelitis.)

|Sinograms (by injection or packing) can detect extension of an ulcer into bursae and/or joint spaces.

|Other imaging studies may be indicated for evaluation of the chest, especially if the source of infection remains in question.

|Bone biopsy (submitted for histological and microbiologic evaluation) is most helpful in confirming the diagnosis of bone infection.

Management

|Management of pressure sore emergencies can be divided into general and local care.

General care:

I. In the case of septic shock, a patient should be monitored in an intensive care unit.

II. Fluid replacement is important because the patient is usually volume-depleted to maintain adequate tissue perfusion. This is usually done with saline solution under guidance of urinary output and pulmonary wedge pressure. Blood or any of its constituents (plasma, albumin, dextran—the latter may cause hemorrhage) may be needed depending on circumstances.

III. Correction of acid-base abnormalities. If the pH is less than 7.1, then small amounts of bicarbonate may have to be given.

IV. Electrolyte imbalances have to be corrected according to the blood chemistry report.

V. Respiratory support is needed for many patients with SCI, especially those with high lesions. Intubation with or without tracheostomy was needed in a high percentage of patients with septic shock.

VI. The sick patient with SCI needs great attention to skin care, bowel care, and catheter care. The nutritional status should be observed as well. The undernourished, confined patient is very susceptible to developing more pressure sores, thus further complicating the situation. Special beds may help to prevent the development of other pressure ulcers. Enteral or parenteral feeding is usually needed.

VII. Sympathomimetic drugs are not safe because of severe vasoconstriction and cardiac irritability. Corticosteroids are controversial. Heparin is rarely indicated because of coagulopathy. Bleeding patients may have replacement therapy, platelet transfusion, and cryoprecipitate or fresh frozen plasma.

VIII. Antibiotic treatment must be specific and adequate. This requires as much information as possible regarding the extent and bacteriologic cause of the infection. Once antibiotic therapy has been initiated, all further microbiologic work-up, i.e., cultures, may be impaired. Therefore, as many cultures and other tests must be submitted prior to starting antibiotics. The more certain of the diagnosis, the more narrow and directed the antibiotic therapy can be. Narrow-spectrum antibiotics translate into less toxicity, less cost, and less chance of inducing resistance in the natural flora.

Table I **Empiric Antibiotic Therapy**
for Infected Decubitus Ulcers with Suspected Bacteremia

Piperacillin-tazobactam or ticarcillin-clavulanate
+/-
gentamicin, tobramycin, or amikacin
+/-
vancomycin

|Table I shows our initial empiric antibiotic regimen for infected decubitus ulcers in patients with suspected bacteremia. An extended-spectrum penicillin with a beta-lactamase inhibitor, such as piperacillin-tazobactam or ticarcillin-clavulanate, provides anti-staphylococcal (except for methicillin-resistant *Staphylococcus aureus* [MRSA]), anti-streptococcal, anti-anaerobic and broad Gram-negative coverage. In the seriously ill patient, an aminoglycoside should be added initially to provide coverage for multi-resistant Gram-negative bacteria until antibiotic sensitivities are known. Toxicity is unusual with 1 or 2 days of aminoglycoside therapy. Vancomycin should be part of the initial antibiotic regimen for patients suspected of being bacteremic in hospitals where there is a significant incidence of MRSA.

Table II **Recommended Antibiotic Therapy**
for Infected Decubitus Ulcers with Suspected Bacteremia

Organism	Antibiotic of Choice (and alternatives)
Streptococcus species (not *Enterococcus*)	Penicillin G or ampicillin (cefazolin, vancomycin, clindamycin)
Enterococcus	Penicillin G or ampicillin or vancomycin plus gentamicin
Enterococcus faecium (VRE)	Linezolid or quinupristin/dalfopristin[1 5]
Staphylococcus aureus (not MRSA)	Nafcillin or oxacillin (cefazolin, piperacillin-tazobactam, or ticarcillin-clavulanate)
MRSA	Vancomycin
Staphylococcus epidermis	Vancomycin[1 5] (unless it is known to be sensitive to nafcillin, oxacillin, or penicillin)
Escherichia coli *Proteus mirabilis*	Cefotaxime or piperacillin-tazobactam, or ticarcillin-clavulanate (aztreonam, aminoglycoside,[1] or quinolone[2])
Serratia marcescens	Cefepime or ceftazidime plus aminoglycoside[1] (imipenem-cilastatin or meropenem)
Anaerobes	Metronidazole or piperacillin-tazobactam or ticarcillin-clavulanate

[1] Aminoglycoside = amikacin, gentamicin, or tobramycin   [2] Quinolone = ciprofloxacin or levofloxacin

|After a specific organism is identified from a blood or wound culture, a more narrow spectrum antibiotic can be used.

Table III **Recommended Dosages**

Antibiotic	Intravenous Dosage
Amikacin*	15 mg/kg/day divided q 24, 12, or 8 hours
Ampicillin	1 gm q 6 hours
Aztreonam	1 gm q 8 hours
Cefazolin	1 to 2 gm q 8 hours
Cefepime	1 gm q 12 hours
Cefotaxime	1 gm q 8 hours
Ceftazidime	1 gm q 8 hours
Ciprofloxacin	400 mg q 12 hours
Clindamycin	600 mg q 8 hours
Gentamicin*	1.5 to 2.0 mg/kg/day divided q 24, 12, or 8 hours
Imipenem/cilastatin	500 mg q 6 hours
Levofloxacin	500 mg q 24 hours
Meropenem	1 gm q 8 hours
Metronidazole	500 mg q 6 hours
Nafcillin	1 gm q 4 hours
Oxacillin	1 gm q 4 hours
Penicillin	G 3 MU q 4 hours
Piperacillin-tazobactam	3.375 gm q 6 hours
Ticarcillin-clavulanate	3.1 gm q 6 hours
Tobramycin*	1.5 to 2.0 mg/kg/day divided q 24, 12, or 8 hours
Vancomycin	1 gm q 12 hours

* Must adjust dose in renal impairment and monitor blood urea nitrogen, SCr, and serum peaks and troughs to avoid nephrotoxicity.

|The recommended dosages of various antibiotics for serious bloodstream infections are shown in Table III. Aminoglycoside therapy requires monitoring for nephrotoxicity with blood urea nitrogen and creatinine determinations 2 or 3 times per week.

|If *Candida* is isolated from a blood culture and the source is suspected to be an infected decubitus ulcer, then antifungal therapy with amphotericin should be initiated. If the organism isolated is identified as *Candida albicans*, then fluconazole can be substituted for amphotericin B because of its excellent safety profile and efficacy.

Local care:

I. Necrotic tissue should be debrided. CO_2-laser debridement is advantageous because the lymphatic and venous channels are sealed by laser beam, thus reducing the showering of bacteria into the blood system. Proper drainage is important. Careful irrigation and light packing should be performed frequently. Suction or suction irrigation with normal saline, lactated Ringer's solution, or Daikin's solution may be appropriate.

II. Cellulitis may subside with 1 to 2 weeks of the appropriate antibiotic. If suppuration occurs, an incision and drainage will be required. Antibiotic selection may be guided by the information in Table I.

III. Lymphangitis and lymphangiophlebitis may be treated adequately by antibiotics and elevation. If deep phlebitis is diagnosed or suspected, anticoagulants should be added.

IV. Septic bursitis requires drainage to help resolve the infection. Incision and drainage is preferable to repeated aspiration.

V. Osteomyelitis as a complication of decubitus ulcers generally results from the contiguous spread of infection. Management includes appropriately selected antibiotics for 4 to 8 weeks, along with surgical debridement by partial or total ostectomy, e.g., Girdlestone procedure in the hip.[16] HBO therapy is also used for 30 to 60 days for treating chronic refractory osteomyelitis.[17,18] Use the following indications for performing amputations: limb ischemia; infection of the whole shaft of a single bone; most cases involving the knee and associated with ischemia. In the upper extremity, even in patients with quadriplegia, conservatism is the rule. (See chapter 17 on osteomyelitis.)

VI. Septic arthritis is frequently due to extension from the pressure sore or from an infected bone. We have seen a few cases in which it was induced by debridement of a pressure sore that is over an open-joint capsule, especially of the knee and ankle. Incision and drainage, along with antibiotics for 4 to 6 weeks, is recommended. Suction irrigation with an antibacterial solution has been used as an alternative. HBO, reconstructive surgery, or amputation may be indicated.

Conclusion

|Pressure sores can lead to serious and even fatal complications, and therefore require prompt attention and aggressive management. Collaborative efforts through different disciplines are often necessary in the management of these cases. Evidence of systemic infection or toxicity should be treated empirically as soon as possible.

Abstract

Basic principles:

I. Pressure ulcers may be complicated by serious sepsis.

II. Patients may be compromised by renal, hepatic, or cardiopulmonary disease, diabetes mellitus, poor nutrition, negligence, or suicide attempts.

III. Sepsis may be local with cellulitis, lymphangitis, arthritis, osteomyelitis, septic phlebitis, or general with septicemia.

IV. In ischemic extremities, gangrene may be manifested.

V. Perineal decubiti may be complicated by necrotizing fasciitis (Fournier's gangrene).

VI. Hemorrhage from a decubitus ulcer may rarely be an emergency.

VII. Autonomic dysreflexia may be a manifestation.

Diagnosis:

I. History of chills or fever (excluding other sources of sepsis, especially urinary tract infection).

II. Signs of local infection: edema, redness, induration, necrosis and tissue gangrene, purulent drainage, or involvement of deeper structures, such as bone or joint.

Management:

I. Bed rest with routine turning, preferable on a special bed.

II. Start IV infusion.

III. Take wound, blood, and urine C&S, aerobic and anaerobic, and Gram stain.

IV. Start therapy depending on the degree of sepsis using 2 or 3 antibiotics (Table I).

V. X-rays if needed.

VI. Local wound care: dressings with or without debridement.

VII. If the patient is in septic shock, transfer to intensive care unit.

VIII. Bleeding from decubiti may be controlled by packing, forcipressure, ligation, or silver nitrate cauterization.

IX. Patient may be taken to the operating room if bleeding persists or for extensive debridement or I&D of abscess.

X. Refer the patient to the SCI surgeon by STAT consultation.

References

1. Young LS. Sepsis Syndrome. In: *Principles and Practice of Infectious Diseases*, Mandell GL, Bennett JE, and Dolin R. Churchill Livingstone: New York, 1995: pp. 690-705.

2. Galpin JE, Chow AW, Bayer AS, et al. Sepsis associated with decubitus ulcers. *Am J Med* 1976;61:346-350.

3. Bryan CS, Dew CE, Reynolds KL, et al. Bacteremia associated with decubitus ulcers. *Arch Int Med* 1983;143:2093-2095.

4. Glenchm H, Patel BS, Pathmarajah C. Transient bacteremia associated with debridement of decubitus ulcers. *Military Med* 1981;146:432-433.

5. Peroment PA, Labbe M, Yourassowsky E, et al. Anaerobic bacteria isolated from decubitus ulcers. *Infection* 1973;1:205-207.

6. Reese RE. Bacteremias and sepsis. In: Reese RE, Douglas Jr G (Eds). *A Practical Approach to Infectious Diseases*. Little Brown & Co.: Boston, Toronto, 1983; pp. 51-162, 181-212.

7. Rissing P, Crowder JG, Dunfee T, et al. Bacteroides bacteremia from decubitus ulcers. *South Med J* 1974:67:1179-1182.

8. Cruse JM, Lewis RE, Bishop GR, et al. Neuro-endocrine immune interactions associated with loss and restoration of immune system function in spinal cord injury and stroke patients. *Journal Res* 1992;11(2):104-116.

9. Segal JL, Gonzales E, Yousefi S, et al. Circulating levels of IL-2R, ICAM-a and IL-6 in spinal cord injury patients. *Arch Phys Med Rehab* 1997;78:44-47.

10. Segal JL. Spinal cord injury: are interleukins a molecular link between neuronal damage and ensuing pathobiology? *Perspectives in Biology and Medicine* 1993;36(2):222-239.

11. Sugarman B, Hawes S, Musher DM, et al. Osteomyelitis beneath pressure sores. *Arch Int Med* 1983;143:683-688.

12. Eltorai I, et al. Urinary Fistulae after radical ischcectomies in surger of ischial pressure sores. *Paraplegia* 1985;23:379-385.

13. Hall PA, Young JV. Autonomic hyperreflexia in spinal cord injured patients. Trigger mechanism—dressing changes of pressure sores. *J Or Trauma* 1983;23(2):1074-1075.

14. Sapico FL, Ginunas VJ, Thronhill-Joynes M, et al. Quantitative microbiology of pressure sores in different stages of healing. *Diagn Microbio Infect Dis* 1986;5:31-38.

15. Moellering RC, Linden PK, Reinhardt J et al. The efficacy and safety of quinupristan/dalfopristan for the treatment of infections caused by vancomycin-resistant *Enterococcus faecium*. *Jour Antimicrobial Chemo* 1999;44, 251-261.

16. Eltorai I. Hyperbaric oxygen in the management of pressure sores in patients with injuries to the spinal cord. *J Dermatol Surg Oncol* 1981;7(9):737-740.

17. Eltorai I. The Girdlestone procedure in spinal cord injured patients: a ten-year experience. *J Amer Paraplegia Soc* 1983;6(4):85-86.

18. Eltorai I, Hart GB, Strauss MB. Osteomyelitis in the spinal cord injured, a review and preliminary report on the use of hyperbaric oxygen therapy. *Paraplegia* 1976;22:17-24.

So-Called
MINOR BURNS Robert E. Montroy, MD, FACS
in Patients With Spinal Cord Dysfunction
CHAPTER NINETEEN ▌

|Minor burns represent the vast majority (95%) of thermal injuries in this country and rarely require hospitalization, as most are superficial with limited morbidity.[1] Most partial-thickness (PT) minor burns heal in 2 to 3 weeks by the regeneration of epithelium and leave no significant scarring. However, deep PT dermal wounds, healing by secondary intention, may develop scar tissue and skin depigmentation. If healing is unduly prolonged over weeks or months or if healing is interrupted by repeated trauma, they may develop unsightly hypertrophic scar tissue. Unfortunately, in susceptible patients, even well-treated minor burns may lead to keloid formation, a condition that differs from a hypertrophic scar in that the scar tissue invades the surrounding normal skin. Another untoward outcome is a PT wound that converts to a full-thickness (FT) skin loss through infection. If such a wound fails to heal or heals slowly by secondary intention over months or years, these chronic wounds are susceptible to malignant degeneration, a condition known as a Marjolin's ulcer.

|The role of the interventionist is to reduce morbidity and promote rapid healing with minimal scarring by the avoidance of inappropriate wound care and by modifying the various intrinsic and extrinsic factors that delay wound healing (Table I). The main effort is to prevent a superficial burn from being converted to an FT wound through infection or secondary trauma, a complication that may require surgical intervention.

|Most patients with minor burns can be successfully treated as outpatients. Patients with spinal cord dysfunction, however, because of a number of biological, socioeconomic, and other factors, are admitted to a spinal cord injury (SCI) unit for the management of their wound. Such a protocol differs from that used to treat the general population where, as one author put it, "We have the philosophy of care that minor burn injuries are similar to abrasions and should be treated as such."[1]

|There is mounting evidence from recent studies that patients with SCI have a compromised immune system with a resultant increased susceptibility to infection.[2-4] This dysfunction involves both humoral and cellular immunity mechanisms with impaired neutrophil phagocytosis, depressed T-cell function, and depressed natural killer cell cytotoxicity. Although not completely understood, the most plausible explanation is that this immune dysfunction is attributed to decentralization of the autonomic nervous system and the loss of supraspinal nervous system control.[2,3] Other medical co-morbidities affecting the immune system, such as diabetes mellitus, compound the risk of developing an infection in a minor wound that is soon converted to an FT wound that may require a skin graft for repair.

Definitions

|The terms of "partial-thickness" burn and "full-thickness" burn have generally replaced the time-honored terms of "first," "second," and "third" degree burns. Such a definition incorporates the concept of treatment, because a PT burn normally can be expected to heal by secondary intention with scar-epithelium, whereas an FT burn connotes the need for a skin graft and healing by primary intention.

|PT burns can be further classified into "superficial" and "deep" PT burns. The deep PT burn destroys epidermis and most of the dermis, leaving only a few dermal cells and the cells of deep epithelial skin appendages, such as the sebaceous and sweat glands, and of the bulb of hair follicles, the residue of which remains in the superficial adipose tissue. These survivor epithelial cells will regenerate (mitosis) and migrate under the stimulus of inflammatory-induced cytokines (growth factors) and are capable of healing a small wound in 4 to 6 weeks by secondary intention.

|The classic way to distinguish a minor burn from a major one relates to the depth of the damaged tissue, as previously stated, and the percentage of the total body surface area (TBSA) involved. Burns of some anatomic sites may be of a limited size compared to the TBSA, yet because of their essential functional role and the potential for functional or cosmetic morbidity, are considered more major injuries, requiring hospitalization in keeping with the guidelines of the American Burn Association.[5]

|The American Burn Association defines a minor burn as a thermal insult causing a cutaneous injury in an adult that is less than 15% (child 10%) of the TBSA with the exception of burns involving the hands, feet, face, and ears, or perineum.[5] FT burns of 2% or more of the TBSA should be treated as inpatients. Age and significant co-morbidities also influence the severity of any burn.

|The TBSA area involved is usually estimated either using body surface area (BSA) charts, such as the Lund and Browder Chart, or the well-known "Rule of Nines," a less accurate but workable method.[6,7] All areas involved in the injury are included in the estimate, both PT and FT burn tissue. Estimating the burned surface area in a minor burn is less complicated and can be done by using the size of the patient's hand as a rough estimate where the palmar surface is approximately 1% of the TBSA.[8]

|The initial estimation of the depth of the burn is more difficult and clinically it is difficult to differentiate between deep PT and FT burns. The time-honored pin prick test for sensory loss in the deep burn, though not without its shortcomings, is of no value in the patient who is paralyzed and already lacking in sensory perception. In the era of early excision and grafting (autograft, homograft, heterograft, or allograft in cases of major burns), trying to differentiate between a deep PT burn and an FT burn may be a moot point in a minor burn, particularly if excision and primary closure is feasible.

|Another way to differentiate between minor and major burns is to consider the molecular and cellular response to an injury. In the major burn, there is a significant general systemic inflammatory reaction in tissues remote from the site of the wound. As part of the body's biological defense mechanisms and the wound-healing process, this generalized inflammatory response is capable of inducing substantial tissue injury of itself. Such a systemic response is not seen in the "minor" injury where the inflammatory response is localized to the injured tissue itself. In order to limit the adverse effects of an uncontrolled inflammation, there is a protective counter-response called forth to regulate and control this acute inflammatory cascade.

|This secondary response in a major burn results in a very "sick patient" (burn "shock,") who requires significant interventions in order to preserve "life and limb," a condition not clinically apparent in minor burns. Although the major thermal injury is perceived as involving only one organ (the integument), the total organism is affected as the anti-inflammatory forces are overwhelmed resulting in the septic inflammatory response syndrome (SIRS).[9] Multi-organ failure can result with severe morbidity and even death.

The Patient With Spinal Cord Dysfunction

|Neurologically impaired individuals, whether their impairment is secondary to trauma or disease, are subject to soft-tissue injuries and wounds from the same variety of causes as the person with an intact nervous system. However, a wound that would be considered trivial or minor in the latter population may have more serious consequences in the patient who, though in good health, has a significant neurological deficit. Although minor in terms of size, depth, and systemic reaction, these so-called minor burns should be viewed in a more serious way in the patient who is paralyzed, where skin integrity is always a major economic and health care concern. These wounds, like pressure sores, if not taken seriously can result in considerable morbidity and in our experience are best treated in the hospital or a skilled nursing facility setting.

|Some of the modifiers that influence our decision-making in this patient population are: 1) compromised socioeconomic conditions, 2) choices in lifestyle, 3) inadequate nutrition, 4) a high bacterial burden of the genitourinary (GU) tract, 5) concomitant pressure sores, and 6) the multiple effects of the neurological deficit, including the difficulties in carrying out the activities of daily living.

|In that many patients with SCI have a limited income due to their disability, or are divorced or widowed, and lack adequate insurance, they are unable to obtain the full-time assistance of a second party needed to help them perform the many activities of daily living. But even with an aide or family member, many of our patients need more than one person to safely turn them every 2 hours in order to avoid imposing an additional friction injury on their "minor" burn. In addition, it is more difficult for a patient in a wheelchair to travel to a medical facility for clinic treatment, particularly if their residence is at a distance from their medical care facility.

|Some of the circumstances surrounding the occurrence of a so-called minor burn in patients with a neurodeficit are not normally encountered by patients with an intact protective sensory nervous system. Prolonged contact with hot water bottles and electric heating pads and driving without protective shoes where there is indirect contact through the floor of the vehicle with the hot muffler/exhaust system are rare occurrences but do happen. In addition, cases of severe sunburn with PT and even FT skin loss that require skin grafting have been reported in sensory-deprived patients who did not perceive the danger signal of skin discomfort while "soaking up good ol' sol" (Figure I).[10]

|A not uncommon scenario is the scald burn where the patient who is wheelchair-bound accidentally spills hot coffee or soup in his/her lap and sustains a scald burn of the thighs and genitalia. In that there is no warning pain involved with absent afferent sensory and efferent motor pathways, the patient does not respond reflexively to the noxious stimulus. In addition, the patients are often physically incapable of quickly removing the super-heated clothing that is in close contact with their skin. Thus, there is prolonged contact with the skin by the hot object resulting in deeper tissue destruction because temperature x time of contact (Injury = T x T) is the formula for the quantity of tissue injured.[11] In addition, the patient frequently may not seek early medical treatment, considering the burn as "minor" until the odor of necrotic and infected tissue gives evidence of a more serious injury.

|The patient who has tetraplegia is more apt to suffer such injuries because of a number of factors that are related to his neurodeficit. The sensory deficit prevents the warning of an injurious event, e.g., the hot beverage taken in a metal cup and burning the hand, the burning cigarette between the distracted patient's fingers. Because of a motor weakness of the upper extremities, a poor handgrip places this patient at risk for losing control of his hot beverage. Spasticity is another factor adversely affecting motor competence and coordination. The use of prosthetic devices and splints used to aid hand motor movements may improve hand function, but not to the degree needed for the patient to handle a full cup of hot liquid.

Management Goals
|The creation of a healthy, healing, wound environment is essential. Constant vigilance for the prevention of infection and the aggressive treatment of an established infection is mandatory. As previously noted, the only acceptable outcome in treating minor burns is a healed wound within an expected and appropriate time frame. Additional goals are the minimizing of cosmetic disfigurement and the prevention of functional impairment secondary to scar formation with tissue contractures.

|All too often these goals are circumvented by the development of the complication of burn wound infection. In the patient with SCI with a neurogenic bladder requiring an indwelling catheter or with a pressure sore, there is a significant bacterial burden present. In addition, the upper thigh/genital or perineal burn wound is at risk from fecal contamination due to the proximity of the terminus of the gastrointestinal tract. Once a PT burn wound becomes infected, it is not uncommon for the acute cellular antimicrobial inflammatory response, with its liberated proteolytic enzymes combined with the released bacterial toxins, to cause the destruction of the remaining viable skin elements leading to an FT skin loss.

Wound Management

|The normal response to a burn incident is to eliminate the heat source as rapidly as possible. In the unattended patient who is paralyzed, this may not be possible, and accounts for the increased severity of this injury in this patient population. If removal of searing wet clothing, as in a scald burn, cannot rapidly be accomplished, then countering the heat with cold water is a reasonable alternative. The use of cold water itself as the initial therapy of the burn, however, is questionable in that after the initial cooling of the burned tissue, prolonged hypothermia may have its own adverse effects on the wound. The prolonged use of ice or ice water in direct contact with the burned surface is not appropriate, as the effects of a cold injury are now added to the equation.

|The cause and circumstances of the injury is usually apparent and is important in the initial assessment, as is the past history of allergies, present medications, and significant illnesses such as diabetes. Pain management is usually not required in the patient with insensate skin, but tetanus prophylaxis is indicated if the patient has not had a booster in the past 5 years.

|The burn site is evaluated for the size of the involved area and an estimate of its depth is made, as it is the basis for the plan of care. Blisters are usually opened, unless the burn involves thick palmar or plantar skin, as blisters are easily broken in the day-to-day care of the patient who is paralyzed. Any intact blisters should be carefully observed for the development of purulent fluid under the intact epithelium and/or an expanding zone of inflammation that would suggest early infection.

|Should the wound be an obvious FT injury of greater than 3 cm, primary excision and the application of a split-thickness skin graft (STSG) may significantly expedite the healing process, barring complications. Skin grafting, however, adds an additional PT wound with its own potential wound-healing complications. The management of STSG donor sites is often more difficult in patients with SCI than the grafted wound itself. It has been have observed in patients with SCI that a high rate of secondary infection develops in the healing donor wound. In addition, the subsequent de-epithelialization by abrasion of the healed but fragile donor site can occur weeks or months later due to presumed shear and other traumatic forces. As a result, it is important to harvest the graft from a sensate donor site above the level of injury, if possible, and from an area not exposed to the pressures of a patient who is bed-bound. An additional option is to take the graft from an area where excision and primary closure of the donor wound is possible. Although synthetic skin substitutes are used in grafting major burns, they are usually not cost-effective in treating minor burns.

|With this experience, these wounds are usually managed medically with a topical antibiotic. Systemic (IV or IM) antibiotics are usually not indicated, as they do not penetrate devitalized tissue that is devoid of circulation, but may be considered in patients with artificial valves, pacemakers, or other internal prosthetic devices. The wound is cleansed with isotonic saline with possibly a mild detergent added as needed. Broken and intact blisters are debrided.

|In that most patients have deep PT injuries when first seen and frequently develop wound infections with multiple organisms (usually Gram-negative), the twice-daily application of the topical antimicrobial cream silver sulfadiazine 1% (Silvadene — Marion Merrill Dow) in non-allergic patients may prevent the progression to a FT wound. Although silver sulfadiazine has been shown to retard wound healing, in the early phase of progressive tissue destruction and tissue invasion by bacteria (infection) the benefits of its broad antimicrobial spectrum outweighs its drawbacks. With the completion of wound debridement, the control of tissue infection, and the initiation of the cellular proliferation phase of wound healing, sulfadiazine is discontinued and the promotion of a moist physiologic wound environment is instituted using appropriate wound-dressing materials. The use of antiseptics, such as 10% povidone iodine solution (Betadine — Purdue Frederick), is avoided because they are toxic to the marginally viable surviving skin cells.

|Because the patient with SCI may be bedridden, careful attention to skin hygiene is important. Avoidance of fecal and/or urinary contamination and being watchful for intertriginous mycotic infections in the groin and genital areas are important. Daily bathing with a bactericidal skin cleanser, such as 4% chlorhexidine gluconate (Hibiclens—Stuart Pharm.) or povidone iodine skin cleanser for its antifungal effects, is important. Good wound care with sterile gloves is necessary. Any concomitant pressure sores with infected necrotic tissue should be appropriately treated.

Education and Prevention

|In that "an ounce of prevention is worth a pound of cure" and "most accidents are preventable," repetitive education of patients, their caregivers, and care providers is obligatory. Reducing the incidence of these so-called minor burns and their attendant morbidity should be a measure of quality improvement. Patients who have experienced one of these "minor" burns become a graduate of the "school of hard knocks" and completely understand the need for avoidance of potential injury situations. Others less heedful need to be cautioned, instructed, and even admonished if noted to be placing themselves in an at-risk position. If a patient in a wheelchair desires to wheel around with a hot cup of coffee in his hand, then a protective water-impervious material, such as a CHUX, is essential. Wheelchairs should have cup holders attached as an additional precaution. All patients with uncontrolled spasms should be assisted when consuming hot liquids.

Conclusion

|The practitioner who is called upon to treat a small burn in a patient with spinal cord dysfunction needs to be aware that the patient is compromised and that any thermal injury may not be minor or trivial and can lead to prolonged morbidity. The injury is usually deeper, takes longer to heal, and is highly susceptible to infection that may require an expensive and extended healing time with all its associated morbidities.

Table I **Factors Adversely Influencing Wound Healing**

Infection	Foreign body
Local toxins/disinfectants	Radiation
Mechanical trauma	Smoking
Vascular insufficiency	Age
Suppression/absence of inflammatory response	Uremia
Malignancy	Alcoholism
Malnutrition	Chemotherapy
Diabetes/metabolic diseases	Jaundice/liver failure
Steroids	Hereditary diseases
Free oxygen radicals	Catabolic metabolism

Figure I

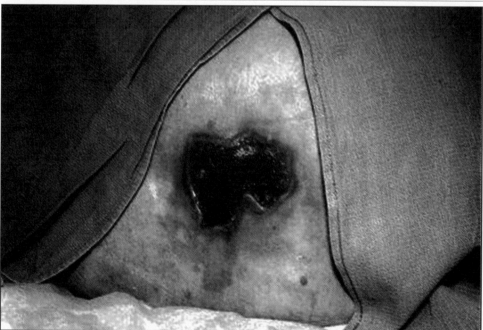

A 70-year-old male with full-thickness skin loss secondary to "minor" burn following the application of hot towels to back by his chiropractor.

References

1. Warden G. Outpatient care of thermal injuries. *Surg Clin NA* 1987;67(1):147-157.

2. Nash MS. Known and plausible modulators of depressed immune functions following spinal cord injuries. *J Spinal Cord Med* 2000;23(2):111-120.

3. Campagnol DI, Bartlett JA, Keller SE. Influence of neurological level on immune function following spinal cord injury: a review. *J Spinal Cord Med* 2000;23 (2):121-128.

4. Cruse JM, Keith JC, Bryant ML Jr, Lewis RE Jr. Immune system-neuroendocrine dysregulation in spinal cord injury. *Immunol Res* 1996;15(4):306-314.

5. American Burn Association Injury Severity Grading System, 1976.

6. Lund CC, Browder NC. Estimation of areas of burns. *Surg Gynecol Obstet* 1944;79:352-358.

7. Polaski GR, Tennison AC. Estimation of the amount of burned surface area. *JAMA* 1934;103:34.

8. Sheridan R, Petras L, Basha G, et al. Should irregular burns be sized with the hand or the palm: a planimetry study. *Proc Am Burn Assoc* 1995;27:262.

9. Bone RC. Systemic inflammatory response syndrome: a unifying concept of systemic inflammation In: *Sepsis and Multiorgan Failure.* (Eds). Fein, MA, Abraham, EM, et al.,Williams Wilkins: Baltimore, 1997.

10. Chung BS, Eltorai I, Furnas D. Thermal injury on the foot and ankle of a paraplegic: report of a case from exposure to sunshine. *J Dermatol Surg Oncol* 1978;4:468-469.

11. Moritz, AR. Studies of thermal injury II: the relative importance of time and surface temperature in causation of cutaneous burns. *Am J of Path* 1947;23:695.

Anousheh Behnegar, MD;
Marcalee Sipski, MD

|MANAGEMENT OF PREGNANCY
in Women With Spinal Cord Disorders and Injuries
CHAPTER TWENTY

|An estimated 3,000 American women of childbearing age per year sustain spinal cord injuries (SCIs) and another significant number of women sustain spinal cord disorders (SCDs) as a result of anatomical anomalies and/or infectious and surgical etiologies.[1] Although most of the research pertaining to pregnancy is related specifically to SCIs, the overall management concepts should be transferrable regarding the management of SCDs. Thus, for purposes of discussion throughout this chapter, when appropriate, the more general term SCDs will be used rather than SCIs.

|It is clear that the development of an SCD is a traumatic and life-changing event that results in a myriad of physical consequences in addition to significant psychological stress. Pregnancy is also a challenging event with subsequent physiologic and psychological changes. Taken together the two conditions need to be judiciously managed to avoid the numerous possible complications. It, therefore, becomes necessary to have a thorough understanding of the effects of SCDs on the reproductive system and pregnancy.

|Twenty years ago, many women with SCDs were cautioned against pregnancy; however, it is now well known that women with SCD are able to give birth with a favorable outcome for mother and baby.[2] Despite this fact, the rate of pregnancy post-SCD remains low. A recent multicenter study reported that only 14% (101 pregnancies) of 472 women became pregnant after SCDs.[3] Similarly, another study revealed a rate of 0.34 pregnancy per woman post-SCD.[4] Because less than 1 per 1,000 pregnancies involve women with SCDs, there is scant clinical information on the management of pregnancy in women with SCD and the interest among clinicians is also limited.[1] Moreover, there are significant deficits in knowledge among internal medicine and OB/GYN residents about management of pregnant women with disabilities and the potential disability-related medical complications of pregnancy.[5] It is hoped that these knowledge deficits will be remediated by training more clinicians and investigators about issues pertaining to women with SCD. Furthermore, as a result of the increased education in this area, it is anticipated that the outlook for successful reproductive function in women with SCDs will continue to improve.

|To be accurate and thorough any discussion of pregnancy in women with SCD must include two distinctly separate categories: the pregnant woman who sustains an SCD and the woman with SCD who becomes pregnant.

Medical Problems of Pregnant Women With SCD

|As the population of women with SCDs of childbearing age increases, so does the need for better understanding of the specific complications they are prone to and their effect on their reproductive ability. Pregnancy in this population of women can be accompanied by many serious medical problems related to their SCD, such as autonomic dysreflexia and urinary tract infections (UTIs). Moreover, a number of these complications, e.g., UTIs, anemia, and deep venous thrombosis (DVT), are also experienced by ambulatory pregnant women.[2]

|Practitioners who are managing pregnant women with SCDs should also pay particular attention to the fact that many of these women are taking a variety of medications in association with their SCDs. The potential effect of these medications on the fetus needs to be recognized and necessary adjustments made in order to safeguard their baby's health. Table I outlines the impact on pregnancy of some medications commonly used in women with SCDs.[2] Because medications are constantly changing, the physician must confirm the safety and need for each medication in the pregnant woman. Consideration should be given to the use of medications that do not cross the placenta in order to minimize the risk of fetal complications. Finally, the pregnant woman with SCD must also be counseled about the dangers of alcohol and tobacco use during pregnancy.

Autonomic Dysreflexia

|Autonomic dysreflexia is a life-threatening condition that occurs in up to 85% of pregnant women with SCDs. Autonomic dysreflexia is characterized by a massive and unrestrained sympathetic outflow in response to sensory stimuli in patients with SCD at or above the T6 level.[1,2,6,7] Though dysreflexia is seen mostly in patients with the lesion at T6 and above, it has also been known to occur in patients with lower thoracic lesions.[2] Practically any stimuli below the lesion, such as increased pressure in the abdominal cavity or dilation of viscera, can precipitate a response.[8,9] The offending stimuli that can trigger autonomic hyperreflexia in pregnancy include distention of bladder, cervix, or rectum, which initiates massive afferent sympathetic and parasympathetic signals without the benefit of modulatory action of the higher control centers.[7,9,10] Signs and symptoms of autonomic dysreflexia range from piloerection, diaphoresis, flushed skin, mild hypertension, headache, and bradycardia to severe hypertension, cerebrovascular accident, cerebral hemorrhage, seizures, pulmonary edema, and death.[7,11-14]

|Autonomic hyperreflexia can occur in the antepartum, intrapartum, and postpartum periods.[2] One study reported an episode triggered by the discomfort of episiotomy. It is important to consider the more common obstetrical hypertensive complication of preeclampsia in the differential diagnosis, the treatment of which is very different than that of autonomic hyperreflexia. The symptoms of dysreflexia, such as hypertension, seem to appear simultaneously with labor contractions in patients with autonomic hyperreflexia, as opposed to eclampsia, where labor pains are usually absent.[1,2,7,12] Prevention, rather than attempts to treat the crisis, is the best way to manage autonomic dysreflexia.[8,12] Gentle cervical exams and effective emptying of bladder and bowel can reduce the risk of dysreflexia.[1,7] Topical anesthetic jelly should be applied before Foley catheter placement or rectal manipulation to reduce afferent activity. The most effective preventive and therapeutic approach to autonomic hyperreflexia in labor and delivery is thought to be regional anesthesia, generally by means of continuous epidural anesthesia.[1,2,7,11,15] The pharmacologic agents commonly used include ganglionic blockers, as well as alpha sympathetic blockers and hydralazine.[1,2,16] If the hypertensive crisis of dysreflexia is not successfully prevented or mitigated by regional anesthetics, short-term antihypertensives, such as sodium nitroprusside and nitroglycerin, have been used. However, all attempts should be made to avoid agents, such as ganglionic blockers and nitroprusside, that can cause significant hypotension in pregnant women.[2] In cases where attempts to control the autonomic hyperreflexia have failed, it may be necessary to perform emergency cesarean or operative vaginal delivery after the patient's hypertension is brought under control.[2] (See chapter 1 on autonomic dysreflexia.)

Anemia

|One of the normal physiological changes that occurs during pregnancy is an increased plasma volume by about 150% at term, accompanied by an unmatched, relatively small increase in red cell volume.[1] This mismatched volume increase leads to hemodilution and anemia of pregnancy. In ambulatory women the average normal hematocrit is about 33% in the second and third trimester of pregnancy.[2]

|It was initially thought that anemia would pose a significant threat to pregnant women with SCDs. However, this fear is unfounded. Pregnant women with SCDs have been shown to have a mean hematocrit of 30% to 36%.[2,17] Transfusions rarely have been required despite the presence of iron deficiency anemia in approximately 70% of pregnant women with SCD.[1] Iron supplementation may become necessary in women with hemoglobins of less than 9 g/dL.[2] However, caution must be exercised when this course of action is considered, because of the additional constipating effect of iron in the face of neurogenic bowel and the potential of a dysreflexic response.[1,2] Anemia may also cause fatigue. More importantly, it increases the risk of developing pressure ulcers and the need for transfusion following delivery; therefore severe anemias should be treated early in the course of pregnancy.[2]

DVT and Pulmonary Embolism

|DVT is the underlying cause of pulmonary thromboembolism, which is a major cause of maternal death in the western world.[18-20] Over 50% of all pregnancy-related DVTs occur during the first and second trimesters and the risk is higher during puerperium than antepartum.[21] Aside from the hypercoagulable state of pregnancy, which predisposes women to this condition, venous stasis secondary to immobility presents an additional risk factor in the pregnant SCD population.[2] Other risk factors include age, operative delivery, obesity, oral contraceptive use, and positive personal and/or family history.[18]

|The mere fact that a woman with SCD is pregnant is not sufficient justification for prophylactic anticoagulation therapy. Rather, patients' risk factors have to be assessed on a case-by-case basis, and their pulmonary functions monitored carefully. Although edema is common in the lower extremities of pregnant women, a major change in its presentation justifies diagnostic evaluation of possible thrombosis.[2] Compression ultrasound is used as a first-line diagnostic tool. If, however, the results are not definitive, venography, CT, and MRI should be considered. Ventilation-perfusion scanning should be used as the primary diagnostic test for detecting pulmonary thromboembolism.[20]

|Once it has been established that anticoagulation is necessary, a routine regimen of heparin should be used for both treatment and prophylaxis of deep venous thrombosis.[2,18] Warfarin is to be avoided because it crosses the placenta and is a known teratogen when used in early pregnancy. Furthermore, it can cause bleeding complications in the fetus and/or mother. Heparin, on the other hand, does not cross the placenta and is relatively safer to use. The possible adverse complications associated with heparin use can be minimized by the use of low-molecular-weight heparins and/or insertion of Greenfield filters.[18,22] The treatment of diagnosed venous thromboembolic event is similar to that in the non-pregnant patient. The Consortium for Spinal Cord Medicine *Clinical Practice Guidelines*, published by Paralyzed Veterans of America (PVA), outlines proper management of DVT.

Pulmonary Function

|In patients with SCDs at the level of T12 and above, the higher the level of SCI, the greater the degree of pulmonary compromise. In addition, in patients with lesions above T10, an impaired cough reflex may increase the risk of pulmonary infection.[23] Pregnancy also normally lowers the maternal oxygen reserve due to decreased functional residual capacity, higher oxygen consumption, and A-a gradient of oxygen.[2] Moreover, the workload of labor and delivery may further compromise pulmonary function.

|In patients with SCDs, the strength or weakness of inspiratory and expiratory muscles determines the need for mechanical ventilation. The best determinant of respiratory muscle function is vital capacity and its two components, which are inspiratory capacity and expiratory reserve volume.[24] These measurements will give a clear assessment of respiratory muscle function. Decreased vital capacity is also one of the physiological consequences of pregnancy, and if it falls below 15 ml/kg of body weight, mechanical ventilation should be implemented.[2,3,23] Regardless of the predelivery vital capacity, it is advisable to have a mechanical ventilator available during labor and delivery for patients with SCDs in anticipation of pulmonary compromise.

Bladder and Bowel Management

|Urinary stasis occurs more commonly during pregnancy, and can be associated with ureteral dilation, decreased bladder tone, and emptying. Asymptomatic bacteriuria increases the chance of developing pyelonephritis by 65% in the general population of pregnant women.[2] Women with SCDs are even more susceptible to UTIs and other complications. Reasons include chronic bacteriuria from incomplete bladder emptying and the presence of indwelling catheters and/or stones.[2,25] Health care practitioners can minimize the incidence of UTIs by avoiding indwelling catheters, if possible, and actively reducing residual urine volumes. There is also an increased incidence of urinary incontinence and frequency, which can continue to the postpartum period. In general, urologic management is reported to become more difficult for some. In one study of women with SCDs, 9.1% reported new bladder spasms sufficient to expel their catheter. Furthermore, 27.3% of women on intermittent catheterization had to catheterize more frequently.[3]

|Pyelonephritis poses a threat both to the mother and fetus because it can lead to sepsis and subsequent adult respiratory distress syndrome and can induce premature labor.[1,2] Urine culture rather than simple urinalysis is recommended to screen all pregnant women during their first antenatal visit.[26,27] Antibiotic treatment of asymptomatic bacteriuria can successfully avert most cases of pyelonephritis in pregnant women.[1,2,28] Pyelonephritis must be treated with antibiotics immediately and frequent follow-up urine cultures is advisable for the duration of the pregnancy.[1,2]

|Women with a neurogenic bowel should maintain the same bowel program used prior to pregnancy. However, increased constipation often occurs as a result of decreased gastric motility during pregnancy.[2] It is therefore advisable to ascertain adequate fluid intake as well as consumption of foods high in fiber content. Stool softeners or glycerin suppositories may need to be used in greater quantities.[1] Topical anesthetics should be considered when manual extraction is needed to minimize the risk of autonomic dysreflexia.

Pressure Ulcers

|The incidence of pressure ulcers in pregnant women with SCD is reported to be 30%.[1] This increased risk is attributed to decreased mobility as a result of weight gain and increased dependence, edema in the lower extremities, anemia of pregnancy, as well as inadequate nutrition. In order to prevent pressure sores, pregnant women should be encouraged to maintain a well-balanced diet and to continue with their range of motion and physical therapy exercises, change position frequently, and wear loose-fitting clothing. Patients should also be provided with proper wheelchair padding. Physicians caring for these women need to pay close attention to skin examination (especially the pressure points) as part of their routine prenatal visits.[2] Furthermore, they must aggressively treat pressure ulcers when they occur, paying attention to the possible adverse effects on the fetus of the various medications being considered.

Spasticity

|Although there is a limited amount of information available about spasticity during pregnancy, it has been noted to increase in severity and frequency.[2] In a recent study, 12% of pregnant women reported worsening of their spasticity.[3] Most anti-spasmodic medications, such as baclofen, diazepam, dantrolene, and Zanaflex, have either not been thoroughly studied for their effects in pregnancy or have been known to be harmful to the fetus (Table I).[1,2] Despite this, because severe spastic episodes can lead to dysreflexia and can be potentially life-threatening to the mother, pharmacotherapy should be considered if necessary.

Table I **Impact on Pregnancy of Medications Commonly Used in Spinal Cord Injured Women***

Medication	Pregnancy Issues	Lactation Issues
Baclofen	Teratogenesis—No data in humans; some abnormalities detected in animal models.	0.1% of maternal dose in milk. Considered compatible with breast-feeding by the American Academy of Pediatrics (AAP).
Diazepam	Teratogenesis—Facial clefts in animals; no good evidence of anomalies in humans. Neurobehavioral—Effects noted in rats but not in humans. Fetal—Third trimester chronic use associated with floppy infant syndrome and diazepam withdrawal syndrome.	Diazepam can accumulate in breast-fed infants as well. Repeated use in nursing mothers is not recommended.
Dantrolene	Little data exists; has been given without adverse effects in the peripartum period to prevent malignant hyperthermia.	No data.
Oxybutynin	Teratogenesis—Anomalies seen in animals given doses toxic to the mothers.	No data.
Pseudoephedrine	Teratogenesis—One small study found increased risk of gastroschisis. Medical—The decongestant of choice in pregnancy.	Not associated with adverse effects in newborns. Considered compatible with breast feeding by the AAP.
Phenoxybenzamine	Fetal—Animal evidence of impaired closure of the ductus arteriosus; used in pheochromocytoma in pregnancy with apparent safety.	No data.

Table I Continued **Impact on Pregnancy of Medications Commonly Used in Spinal Cord Injured Women***

Medication	Pregnancy Issues	Lactation Issues
Prazosin	Teratogenesis — Not seen in animals; fetal and maternal toxicity at high doses in animals. Fetal — Used with apparent safety for hypertension in few patients.	No data.
Calcium channel blockers	Teratogenesis — Animal and in vitro evidence of several abnormalities. Fetal — Animal evidence of acid base disturbance. Medical — Used with safety in series of women in third trimester for preterm labor.	Less than 5% of material dose in milk. Nifedipine is considered compatible with breast-feeding by the AAP.
Nitrofurantoin	Teratogenesis — Not seen in animals; fetal and maternal toxicity at high doses in animals. Medical — No reports of fetal hemolytic anemia (theoretically at risk).	Considered compatible with breast-feeding by the AAP unless the child has G6PD deficiency.
Trimethoprim-sulfamethoxazole	Teratogenesis — Anomalies seen in animals; little evidence in humans. Fetal — Concern over displacement of bilirubin from albumin and from impaired folate availability. Teratogenesis — No evidence of anomalies in animals.	Compatible with breast-feeding unless premature, jaundiced, or G6PD deficiency.
Ciprofloxacin	Fetal — Arthropathy in animals; use not recommended in pregnant women.	Not compatible with breast-feeding.

° Reproduced with permission from "Pregnancy in Spinal Cord Injured Women" by Baker.

Management of Women Who Sustain SCI While Pregnant

|Management of a pregnant woman who has been involved in any kind of accident and presents with back pain, neurological changes, and/or impaired consciousness must be geared to minimize further neurological damage by stabilizing the spine as well as maintaining airway and cardiovascular integrity.[1] Sedation and anesthesia should be readily available and administered as needed.[2] If the patient is in the third trimester, an obstetrician should be present in case emergency delivery of the fetus is deemed necessary.[1,2]

|Hypotension can be a serious complication of SCD due to neurogenic shock resulting in vasodilation, increased venous pooling, and decreased cardiac output. Additionally, maternal bradycardia may ensue secondary to loss of sympathetic tone and unopposed parasympathetic activity. Other causes of hypotension include uterine injury as well as placental abruption.[1,2] Intravenous crystalloid infusions and transfusions must be started as soon as possible to correct the hypovolemia. If necessary, pressor agents, such as dopamine, can be used effectively without harmful effects on the fetus.[2]

|The woman's respiratory status must be assessed and necessary steps taken to prevent hypoxemia. Depending on the level of injury, intubation and mechanical ventilation may be required (cervical lesions). Furthermore, injuries to the thoracic spine may cause hypoventilation and respiratory insufficiency due to the damaged nerve supply of intercostal and accessory respiratory muscles.[1]

|If the patient is not in the third trimester, she should lie supine and be moved by log rolling only. In the third trimester, however, a lateral-tilt position is preferred to minimize the risk of aortocaval compression with decreased maternal cardiac output, placental hypoperfusion, and the resulting fetal hypoxemia.[2] The most common cause of fetal death, following a traumatic injury to the mother, is abruptio placenta, which occurs in 5% of women with minor trauma and 50% of women who sustain major trauma.[1,2]

|Hypotension and severe hypoxia have been associated with fetal structural developmental defects in the first trimester and neural tissue damage in the second and third trimesters. In general, mechanical injury to the fetus following maternal trauma is prevented by the cushioning effect of the amniotic fluid. However, if the fetus does sustain injuries, it more commonly involves the skull and long bones.[2] Although ultrasonography is a valuable diagnostic tool to identify fetal abnormalities, patients need to be advised that it does not detect all fetal malformations. Patients should be apprised that the rate of fetal malformations is increased to 3% in the event of SCD.[2]

|When providing medical care to the pregnant woman, one must also consider the impact of diagnostic tests and therapeutic procedures. More than 5 rads of radiation is required to place the fetus at risk for malformation in the first trimester; however, care should be taken to shield the fetus from diagnostic radiation if possible.[2] For example, abdominal and lumbar spine X-rays each expose the fetus to about 300 millirads of radiation. Surgical stabilization of the spine has been shown to be safe and effective in pregnancy. Use of spinal orthotics and whether or not they impede fetal growth should be considered on an individual basis.

|For those pregnant women who sustain SCDs, the need for psychological counseling is paramount to help women cope with significant physical and emotional ramifications of pregnancy and the future of the unborn fetus. These women also need to be counseled by a maternal-fetal medicine specialist on the risk to the fetal development and possible outcome of their pregnancy.[29] Patient and family education are of paramount importance in anticipating and dealing with serious complications.

Labor and Delivery

|There is no evidence of increased risk of stillbirths or birth defects among pregnant women with SCDs.[17] In fact, one report revealed a greater percentage of miscarriages (12.7%) before injury compared to only 6% after injury.[3] However, pregnant women with SCDs face unique complications during labor and delivery and for this reason, attempts must be made to prevent unsupervised delivery.[1,2] This holds true especially in the case of women whose sensations of uterine contractions are uncertain.

|Perception of labor is dependent upon the level and completeness of the spinal cord lesion.[2,30] First-stage labor pain is transmitted by sympathetic fibers entering the spinal cord at T10-L1 and second-stage labor pain signals travel along the pudendal nerve entering the cord at S2-4. Patients with spinal cord lesions below T10 should be able to feel uterine contractions, though the sensations may still be different than that of the ambulatory women. Moreover, most women with SCDs experience labor through vague symptoms, such as abdominal cramping, back pain, leg or abdominal spasms, or symptoms of autonomic hyperreflexia.[2,3] Symptoms of autonomic dysreflexia are an indication for cervical examination.[17]

|Although preterm labor was thought to occur at a much higher rate in women with SCDs, recent studies have shown the rate of preterm labor is only slightly higher than that of the general population of women.[2,17] Another misconception about pregnancy in women with SCD is rapid labor, which can be attributed to the lack of sensation of latent labor in these women.[2] In reality, it has been shown that the duration of labor is very similar to that of ambulatory women. In order to avoid unattended delivery, it is recommended that weekly cervical examinations be performed starting at 28 weeks of gestation.[2,5,14,23] Furthermore, patients should be taught to palpate for uterine contractions to detect preterm labor. Home uterine contraction monitoring may be considered in cases of total inability of the patient to perceive preterm labor.[2,17] The diagnosis of labor is generally confirmed by palpation of contractions and vaginal examination.[1]

|Vaginal delivery is preferred, but obstetrical indications may dictate cesarean delivery. Forceps deliveries or vacuum extractions may be necessary in women with inadequate expulsive ability.[2] Deformed pelvis and the presence of intractable autonomic dysreflexia unresponsive to medication or anesthesia are additional indications for cesarean delivery in women with SCD. The rate of cesarean delivery is reported to range from 20% to 30% in the SCD population as compared to 25% in the ambulatory population.[2,17]

|Postpartum complications include episiotomy dehiscence or infection. These problems can be minimized by frequent perineal cleansing, warm sitz baths, and use of techniques aimed at reducing the chance of tissue necrosis.[2] Vaginal delivery may also cause a permanent deterioration of bladder function. Bladder retention must be avoided by catheterization or non-catheter techniques to prevent UTI and/or dysreflexia. Patients should be monitored carefully for signs of postpartum uterine contractions, because they have been known to trigger autonomic dysreflexia.[2]

Conclusion

|It is reassuring to confirm the belief that childbirth is not only possible but safe after paralysis. With the use of currently available information and by providing thoughtful and coordinated medical care, practitioners can facilitate an uneventful and successful course of pregnancy. More research is needed to study the various complications associated with pregnancy in women with SCDs in order to allow better understanding and treatment of each problem as they arise. The management of the pregnant woman with SCD must be individualized and is best accomplished through a coordinated interdisciplinary approach. Moreover, when childbirth is completed and the woman with SCD must cope with the challenges of motherhood, the need for continued physical and emotional support is paramount. Further research is also needed to understand the needs of mothers with SCDs and their children.

References

1. Attenbury JL, Groom LJ. Pregnancy in women with spinal cord injuries. *Orthopedic Nursing* 1998;33(4):603-611.

2. Baker E R, Cardenas DD. Pregnancy in Spinal Cord Injured Women. *Arch Phys Med Rehab* 1996;77:501-507.

3. Jackson AB, Wadley V. A Multicenter Study of Women's Self-Report Reproductive Health After Spinal Cord Injury. *Arch Phys Med Rehab* 1999; 80:1420-1428.

4. Charlifue SW, Gerhart KA, et al. Sexual issues of women with spinal cord injuries. *Paraplegia* 1992;30:192-199.

5. Oshima, S, Kirschner, KL, Heinemann, A, Semik, P. Assessing the knowledge of future internists and gynecologists in caring for a woman with tetraplegia. *Arch Phys Med Rehab* 1998;79:1270-1272.

6. McGregor, JA, Meeuwsen, J. Autonomic hyperreflexia: a mortal danger for spinal cord injured women in labor. *Am Ob Gyn* 1985;151(3):330-333.

7. Travers PL. Autonomic dysreflexia: a clinical rehabilitation problem. *Rehab Nurs* 1999;24(1):19-23.

8. Karlsson AK, Friberg P, Lonnroth P, et al. Regional sympathetic function in high spinal cord injury during mental stress and autonomic dysreflexia. *Brain* 1998;121(Pt 9):1711-1719.

9. Krenz NR, Meakin SO, Krassioukov AV, Weaver LC. Neutralizing intraspinal nerve growth factor blocks autonomic dysreflexia caused by spinal cord injury. *J Neurosci* 1999;19(17):7405-7414.

10. Verduyn WH. Pregnancy and Delivery in Tetraplegic women. *Spinal Cord Medicine* 1997;20(3):371-374.

11. Karlsson, AK. Autonomic Dysreflexia. *Spinal Cord* 1999;37(6):383-391.

12. Sansone GR, Bianca R, Cueva-Rolon, R Gomez, LE, Komisaruk, BR. Cardiovascular responses to vaginocervical stimulation in the spinal cord-transected rat. *Am J Physiol* 1997;273(4 Pt.2):R1361-R1366.

13. Wanner MB, Rageth, CJ, Zäch GA. Pregnancy and autonomic hyperreflexia in patients with spinal cord lesions. *Paraplegia* 1987;25:482-490.

14. Young BK, Katz M, Klein SA. Pregnancy after spinal cord injury: altered maternal and fetal responses to labor. *Obstet Gynecol* 1983;62(1):59-63.

15. Hughes SJ, Short DJ, Usherwood M.McD, Tebbutt H. Management of pregnant woman with spinal cord injuries. *Br J Obstet Gynecol* 1991;98:513-518.

16. Vaidyanatha S, Soni BM, Sett P, Watt JW, Oo T, Bingley J. Pathophysiology of autonomic dysreflexia: long-term treatment with terazosin in adult and pediatric spinal cord injury patients manifesting recurrent dysreflexic episodes. *Spinal Cord* 1998;36(11):761-770.

17. Baker ER, Cardenas DD, Benedetti TJ. Risks associated with pregnancy in spinal cord injured women. *Obstet Gynecol* 1992;80:425-428.

18. Greer IA. The special case of venous thromboembolism in pregnancy. *Haemostasis* 1998;28(Suppl 3):22-34.

19. Greer IA. Thrombosis in pregnancy: maternal and fetal issues. *Lancet* 1999;353(9160):1258-1265.

20. Macklon NS. Diagnosis of deep venous thrombosis and pulmonary embolism in pregnancy. *Curr Opin Pulm Med* 1999;5(4):233-237.

21. Ray JG, Chan WS. Deep vein thrombosis during pregnancy and the puerperium: a meta-analysis of the period of risk and the leg of presentation. *Obstet Gynecol Surv* 1999; 54(4): 265-271.

22. Aburahma AF, Boland JP. Management of deep vein thrombosis of the lower extremity in pregnancy: a challenging dilemma. *Am Surg* 1999;65(2):164-167.

23. Greenspoon, JS, Paul RH. Paraplegia and quadriplegia: special considerations during pregnancy and labor and delivery. *Am J Obstet Gynecol* 1986;155(4):738-741.

24. Macklem, PT. Muscular weakness and respiratory function. *N Engl J Med* 1986;314(12):775-776.

25. Sipski ML. Spinal cord injury and sexual function: an educational model. *Sexual Function in People with Disability and Chronic Illness*. Aspen Publishers, Inc., Gaithersburg, MD. Editors: Marcal L. Sipski, MD, Craig L. Alexander Ph.D 1997:169-173.

26. Patterson TF, Andriole VT. Detection, significance and therapy of bacteriuria in pregnancy: update in the managed health care era. *Infect Dis Clin NA* 1997;11(3): 93-608.

27. Chongsomchai C, Piansriwatchara E, Lumbiganon P, Pianthaweechai K. Screening for asymptomatic bacteriuria in pregnant women: urinanalysis vs. urine culture. *J Med Assoc Thailand* 1999;82(4):369-373.

28. Faro S, Fenner DE. Urinary tract infections. *Clin Obstet Gynecol* 1998;41(3):744-754.

29. Nygaard I, Bartscht KD, Cole S. Sexuality and reproduction in spinal cord injured women. *Obstet Gynecol Surv* 1990;45(11):727-732.

30. Westgren N, Hulting C, Levi R, Westgren M. Pregnancy and delivery in women with a traumatic spinal cord injury in Sweden. *Obstet Gynecol* 1993;81(6) 926-929.

Suggested Reading

I. Bergman SB, Yarkony GM, Stein SA. Spinal cord injury rehabilitation. 2. Medical complications. *Arch Phys Med Rehab* 1997; 78(3 Suppl): S53-S58.

II. Lechter JC Jr., Goldfine, LJ. Management of a pregnant paraplegic patient in a rehabilitation center. *Arch Phys Med Rehab* 1986;67(7):477-478.

III. Salzberg, CA, Byrne, DW, et al. Predicting and preventing pressure ulcers in adults with paralysis. *Adv Wound Care* 1998;11(5):237-246.

THERMOREGULATION

in Patients With SCI

CHAPTER TWENTY-ONE ▰▰▰

Thomas C. Cesario, MD

Temperature regulation is a process that involves many systems.[1-3] Initially, heat is generated by one of several processes including muscular activity, metabolic events, and digestive processes. The rate of dissipation of the heat generated by these events has a profound influence on body temperature. The regulation of the heat loss from the body establishes body temperature. Both physiological and behavioral factors participate in controlling body temperature. The behavioral factors involve seeking environments that either increase or diminish the rate of heating in order to maintain body temperature within narrow limits.

The physiological mechanisms are more complex. First, both heat and cold signals can be received from skin receptors and constitute the first component of the afferent thermoregulatory system. Heat receptors can be identified in both the skin and the central nervous system. The heat receptors in the preoptic area of the hypothalamus respond to changes in blood temperature and activate other hypothalamic centers. Actual adjustment in body temperature is mediated by the hypothalamus, which receives signals from these centers in the anterior hypothalamus, midbrain, spinal cord, or other areas. The hypothalamus integrates these signals and mounts the appropriate response.

|In addition, endocrine factors may participate in thermal regulation. Thus, decreased secretion of vasopressin may diminish the volume of body fluid to be heated and thus help raise body temperature.

|The mechanisms by which hypothalamic centers accomplish thermal regulation can be mediated through the sympathetic nervous system. Inhibition of the sympathetic nervous system occurs normally from hypothalamic centers if it is perceived that body temperature is too warm, resulting in vasodilation and possibly other cooling measures. Conversely, if it is perceived by the hypothalamus that body temperature is too cool, the sympathetic centers will be excited with subsequent vasoconstrictor and possibly other heat-conserving mechanisms.

|Other mechanisms to increase heat production and help raise or maintain body temperature include shivering (the most potent mechanism), increased cellular metabolism, and, of course, heat-seeking behavior. The shivering mechanism involves afferent mechanisms from cold receptors in the skin, the posterior hypothalamus, and efferent connections with anterior motor neurons in the spinal cord. For cooling, the body may employ sweating, which is also primarily controlled by the hypothalamus and, again, behavior modalities to seek cooler areas. These mechanisms in the normal person are so effective that a normal body temperature can be maintained in environments ranging between 13° C and 60° C.

|Fever itself is often accomplished through the release of endogenous pyrogens.[2,3] These are secreted by a number of different cells in the body, but especially macrophages. Endogenous pyrogens include interleukin 1 beta, interleukin 6, tumor necrosis factor alpha, and interferons beta and gamma. Secretion of these endogenous pyrogens can occur when the appropriate cells (usually macrophages) interact with various substances including microbes, antigen antibody complexes and complement, and certain complement components. Endogenous pyrogens, in turn, travel to the hypothalamus via the bloodstream to change the set point for the body temperature. The brain recognizes endogenous pyrogens in the circumventricular organs that lack the blood brain barrier. Changing the set point is accomplished in the hypothalamus through the use of a number of substances, particularly prostaglandins. However, the final effector pathways for fever must travel over neural pathways to the cutaneous vasculature and shivering mechanisms.

|Because neural pathways are important in the modulation of fever, the question of temperature regulation in the patient with spinal cord injury (SCI) is a relevant one. Patients with complete SCI above T6 usually have difficulty maintaining normal body temperature.[4-12] Such patients exhibit partial poikilothermia with lower core temperatures in the cold, and higher ones in the heat. This inability to maintain a constant core temperature is due to lack of effective afferent pathways from skin receptors and inability to perform vasoconstriction, vasodilation, and sweating in the insentient portion of the body. There is also evidence that patients with SCI may be able to alter the thermal set point dependent on the ambient temperature.[13] There is some evidence that thermoregulatory vasomotor tone may be adjusted through spinal cord reflexes and some investigators have described sweating in persons with quadriplegia. Clearly, wider swings in body temperature may occur in patients with SCI and, thus, these patients should avoid extremes in ambient temperature.

|Based on these considerations of thermal instability in patients with SCI, one might anticipate that the presence of fever is not necessarily as reliable an indicator of infection as in the non-SCI population.[14] Theoretically, patients with SCI should be able to increase body temperature only by shivering and vasoconstricting in areas above the cord interruption; however, fever in these patients is common. Thus, Colachis and Otis reported 60 of 71 patients with acute SCI had fever at least at some point in their hospitalization.[15] Sugerman et al, when studying 72 patients hospitalized on an SCI service after the initial injury (beginning 4 to 6 weeks after injury), reported most patients with fevers had infections.[16] Indeed, only 8 of 71 prospectively surveyed patients and 2 of 106 retrospectively surveyed patients had unexplained fever, and only 1 in the former group, and none in the latter, had autonomic dysreflexia to explain temperature elevations. Beraldo et al reported similar findings.[17] Thus, despite the abnormal thermoregulatory abilities of patients with SCI, elevation of temperature (38° C or more) must always necessitate a careful search for a cause, especially those of an infectious nature.

|Several types of infections are particularly common in patients with SCI. These include respiratory, urinary, and cutaneous infections. Two recent studies have suggested the incidence of atelectasis or pneumonia ranges from 35% to 50% in the acute period following SCI.[18-19] Thus, in the differential diagnosis of fever in this setting, processes occurring in the lung must be considered.

|The most common complication in the early period of rehabilitation after acute SCI is urinary tract infection, and this continues to be a major problem throughout the lives of these individuals.[20] Intermittent self-catheterization as opposed to indwelling catheterization may decrease the occurrence of this complication.

|Finally, infected pressure sores are always a threat for patients with SCI. Prevention, of course, is the best approach to this complication.

Editor's Note

|Because patients with tetraplegia are liable to environmental poikilothermia, it is important to have an adjustable environmental temperature. As previously stated, infection should be ruled out first. From our experience, after exhausting the clinical and laboratory tests for the usual causes of pyrexia, one should still think of infection of some kind somewhere in the body, particularly genitourinary and respiratory infections. Rarely, the source may be undiagnosed for a while, but one should think of occult sites, e.g., septic arthritis of the hip, osteomyelitis, perinephritis, abscesses at injection sites, prostatic abscess, meningioencephalitis, subacute bacterial endocarditis, fecal impaction intoxication, drug fever, etc. With the modern diagnostic techniques, especially ultrasound and CT scans, the source is usually diagnosable.

References

1. Atkins A, Bodel. Fever. *N Engl J Med* 1972;286:27-35.

2. Dinarello C, Wolff S. Pathogenesis of fever in man. *N Engl J Med* 1978;298:607-612.

3. Dinarello C, Cannon J, Wolff S. New concepts on the pathogenesis of fever. *Reviews in Infect Dis* 1988;10:168-189.

4. Downey JA, Chiodi HP, Darling RC. Central temperature regulation in the spinal man. *J Appl Physiol* 1967;22(1):91-94.

5. Downey JA, Huckaba CE, Myers SJ, et al. Thermoregulation in the spinal man. *J Appl Physiol* 1973;34(6):790-794.

6. Downey JA, Huckaba CE, Kelley PS, et al. Seating responses to central and peripheral heating in spinal man. *J Appl Physiol* 1976;40(5):701-706.

7. Guttmann L, Silver J, Wyndham. Thermoregulation in spinal man. *J Appl Physiol* 1958;142:406-419.

8. Guttmann L. *Spinal Cord Injuries: Comprehensive Management and Research*, ed 2. Blackwell Scientific Publications: Melbourne, 1976.

9. Pledger HG. Disorders of temperature regulation in acute traumatic tetraplegia. *J Bone & Joint Surgery* 1962;44-B:110-112.

10. Pembrey MS. The temperature of man and animals after section of spinal cord. *Brit Med J* 1897;2:883-884.

11. Schmidt K, Chan C. Thermoregulation and fever in normal persons and in those with spinal cord injuries. *Mayo Clin Proceedings* 1992;67:469-475.

12. Sherrington CS. Notes on temperature after spinal transection with some observations on shivering. *J of Physiol* 1984;58:405-424.

13. Attia M, Engel T. Thermoregulatory set points in patients with spinal cord injuries (spinal man). *Paraplegia* 1983;21:233-248.

14. Tigay EL. Disregulation of temperature control in cervical spinal cord lesions. Paraplegia Conference, Veterans Administration Hospital, Hines IL, pg. 80.

15. Colachis S, Otis S. Occurrence of fever associated with thermoregulation dysfunction after acute spinal cord injury. *Am J Phys Rehab* 1995;74:114-119.

16. Sugerman B, Brown D, Musher D. Fever and infection in spinal cord injury patients. *JAMA* 1982;248(1):66-70.

17. Beraldo P, Neves E, Alves C, et al. Pyrexia in hospitalized spinal cord injury patients. *Paraplegia* 1993;31:186-191.

18. Fishburn M, Marino R, Ditunno J. Alatetasis and pneumonia in acute spinal cord injury. *Arch Phys Med Rehab* 1990;71:197-200.

19. Reines HD, Harris R. Pulmonary complications of acute spinal cord injuries. *Neurosurgery* 1987;21:193-196.

20. Cardenas D, Mayo M. Bacteriuria with fever after spinal cord injury. *Arch Phys Med Rehab* 1987;68:291-293.

|INFECTIONS

Thomas C. Cesario, MD

in Spinal Cord Injury Patients

CHAPTER TWENTY-TWO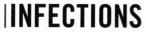

|Patients with spinal cord injury (SCI) are uniquely predisposed to infection by virtue of their lack of mobility, inability to perform bodily functions in a normal manner, and the presence of various tubes inserted into the body through different portals. The risk of infection in this setting will vary with the degree of disability and the presence of other factors or conditions that may enhance the frequency of infections. Thus Sugarman et al noted 67% of patients admitted to an SCI service during a 1-year period developed fever or infection.[1] The most common single causes of infection found in this study were related to urinary tract (39% of patients) and soft-tissue infections (17% of patients).

|These authors also evaluated 46 patients retrospectively who had been seen by the infectious disease service. A total of 106 infections were reported in these patients. These included 32 urinary tract infections (UTIs) (31%) and 36 soft-tissue infections (35%). Other causes of fever occurring in the latter, more chronic, group included osteomyelitis (18%) and respiratory tract infections (8%).

|Similarly, Beraldo et al reported on pyrexia in patients with SCI. They studied all new episodes of fever occurring in a 3-month period. They also determined the incidence of fever among these patients to be 33.9 new episodes per 100 patient-months.[2] In only 8% of these cases was no cause found. The most common causes determined were again UTI (44.3%) and soft-tissue infections (11.4%).

|Colachis and Otis also examined the occurrence of fever after acute SCI.[3] They found in a retrospective study spanning a 2-year period that 60 of 71 at-risk patients had fever at some point during the time of the investigation. UTIs were again most common (59 of 141 proven febrile episodes), but respiratory tract infections were the second most frequent type of infections seen (40 of 141 episodes). Soft-tissue infections were less common (5 of 141 proven episodes). The higher incidence of respiratory tract infections and the lower incidence of soft-tissue infections may relate to the acuteness of the injury.

|Because urinary dysfunction is frequent in patients with SCI, it is expected that UTIs will be very common. The first problem warranting consideration in this setting is prevention. Because many of these patients are unable to void, some form of intervention is needed. Most frequently this takes the form of catheter drainage. It is thus accepted in patients with acute SCI that intermittent catheterization is preferable.[4]

|For the long term it is hoped that intermittent catheterization will lead to a time when reflex bladder activity returns. Should this fail, other measures, including Crede maneuvers or suprapubic taping, may be considered. However, chronic intermittent catheterization is still useful, especially if the patient has enough upper extremity function to allow him to perform this task himself. If the patient cannot perform this function and the family is unable to assist, then chronic indwelling catheterization may be used, although there remain many complications from this strategy.

|Finally, the question of chronic clean intermittent catheterization vs. sterile catheterization appears to be resolved by several studies that have suggested appropriately done clean intermittent catheterization has no higher complication rate.[5, 6]

|Bacteriuria in patients with SCI is common whatever technique of bladder emptying is employed. With chronic indwelling catheters virtually all will become bacteriuric. Among those patients with intermittent catheterization, King et al found that among patients admitted to an SCI service, with a mean duration of admission of 60 days, 28 of 46 patients (61%) developed bacteriuria during admission and 20 were symptomatic.[7] The incidence of bacteriuria did not vary with sterile vs. clean catheterization. Thus it is likely that even patients with intermittent catheterization will become bacteriuric. The length of time to bacteriuria likely depends on the care with which the catheter is prepared and inserted.

|Once bacteriuria develops, treatment is usually reserved for symptomatic patients or patients with some special complication. Symptoms would include fever and, of course, any irritative complaints referable to the urinary tract if they can be perceived by the patient. Assurance that the UTI is the cause of the fever, if the fever is the only symptom, is more problematic because bacteriuria alone is so common in these patients. Gross pyuria—greater than 50 white blood cells (WBC) per high power field—has been associated with fever and bacteriuria in patients with indwelling catheters.[8] If patients do not have indwelling catheters, then smaller numbers of cells are significant. What can be particularly useful is a change in pyuria. Thus, knowing the WBC count in the urine during afebrile periods can constitute a useful baseline. On occasion, however, the assumption that a UTI is the cause of fever must be made if no other cause can be found and bacteriuria exists.

|The appropriate antibiotics to treat UTIs in patients with SCI may vary depending on bacterial sensitivities. Because most of these individuals have had exposure to prior antibiotics or have institutionally acquired organisms, it is best to presume the organism is resistant to antibiotics and, therefore, broader-spectrum agents are appropriate until antibiotic sensitivities are available. Thus, quinolones, broad-spectrum beta-lactams, monobactams, and aminoglycosides are appropriate. When antibiotic sensitivities become available, the choice of antibiotic can be altered to something with a narrower spectrum.

|Cutaneous infections are the second most common causes of fever among patients with SCI. These infections include infected pressure ulcers. Pressure sores themselves are common among patients with SCI. Thus Fuhrer reported that 33% of patients with SCI had a pressure ulcer of at least grade-1 severity and 13.6% of patients had one or more stage 3 or 4 pressure ulcers.[9] Further, Sugarman et al reported that 6 of 25 pressure sores in their prospective study became infected.[1] Signs of infection would include fever, spreading erythema, and purulence of the ulcer. Treatment includes debridement, which for the simplest ulcers can be only wet-to-dry dressing changes, but in the more advanced cases will require surgical debridement. Infected pressure ulcers may lead to osteomyelitis as well. Sugarman et al noted this complication in 2 of the 6 patients with infected pressure ulcers.[1] Once infection develops, antibiotics are generally appropriate. Cultures from these sites often show mixed organisms including aerobic Gram-positive and Gram-negative organisms as well as anaerobes. Culture with antibiotic sensitivities again becomes paramount but, in the interim, broad-spectrum coverage is appropriate. Thus agents like ticarcillin/clavulanate, ampicillin/sulbactam, or piperacillin/tazobactam may be used initially but, for more resistant infections, combinations of agents to cover Gram-positive organisms (nafcillin or first-generation cephalosporins), anaerobes (clindamycin or metronidazole), and Gram-negative organisms (quinolones and extended-spectrum beta-lactams, monobactams, or aminoglycosides) must be used. Of course, the best measure to deal with pressure ulcers is prevention.

|Respiratory complications are yet another problem for patients with SCI and can be serious. Cheshire reported 15% to 18% of deaths among patients with SCI in the first 3 months after injury had a pulmonary cause, and Bellamy et al in 1973 suggested 10% of the fatalities in the first year after injury were pulmonary-based.[10,11] Among respiratory complications, atelectasis and pneumonia are most common as reported by Goetter et al and by Reines and Harris.[12,13] Both of these complications are most common in the first 3 weeks post-injury and relate to the degree of respiratory impairment. Thus, patients with quadriplegia have a higher incidence of these problems then do those with paraplegia, according to Fishburn et al, who found that 50% of patients with SCI had either atelectasis or pneumonia in the first 30 days post-injury.[14] To differentiate this further, Reines and Harris reported that among 123 consecutive patients admitted to a neurosurgical service with SCI, there were 53 cases of pulmonary complications (35.7%).[13] These included 24 cases of atelectasis (20%) and 13 cases of pneumonia (11%). Again, the degree of respiratory impairment was directly associated with the risk of these complications.

|Because cases of pneumonia in patients with SCI are likely nosocomial in origin, one must anticipate the likely organisms to be more antibiotic-resistant. Thus hospital-acquired Gram-negative rods must always be considered as potential causes of the problem in the patients with SCI. Aspiration pneumonia with the presence of anaerobic organisms must also be kept in mind. Obtaining adequate specimens for Gram stain and culture is critical to defining appropriate antibiotic regimens. This process of specimen collection may be complicated if cough is impaired and may therefore require tracheal suctioning with trapping of the specimen or bronchoscopy.

|Empiric therapy should include broad-spectrum coverage with single agents if the patient is stable (ticarcillin/clavulanate or imipenem) or combination therapy if the infection is severe. The latter might include such agents as clindamycin, a quinolone, and a third-generation cephalosporin. Other combinations would be equally useful and therapy can be adjusted with return of the cultures.

|Thromboembolism is another potential cause of fever in this setting. Thus the incidence of apparent thromboembolic disease in patients with acute SCI and without anticoagulation has been reported to vary from 12.5% to 40% for deep venous thrombosis and 5% to 13% for pulmonary embolization.[15,16] Weingarden et al has pointed out that this can be associated with fever in the patients with SCI.[17] Clearly, appropriate suspicion and diagnosis with venography, radionuclide scanning, or plethysmography is helpful. Ventilation/perfusion scans of the lung for pulmonary embolism can be most helpful. Appropriate anticoagulation is likely necessary.

|Heterotopic ossification, the formation of bone in abnormal anatomic locations, can be a cause of fever in patients with SCI. This commonly occurs around neurologically affected joints and occurs in 16% to 53% of patients.[18] Tow and Kong have reported the association of prolonged fever with heterotopic ossification.[19] Typically occurring in the first 4 months after SCI, heterotopic ossification commonly presents with swelling, warmth, erythema, and tenderness of involved joints. Indomethacin has been suggested to be prophylactic in the prevention of heterotopic ossification, although this is open to dispute.[19,20] Tow and Kong have reported that indomethacin treatment was associated with termination of fever in their case.[19]

|Other causes of fever include thermoregulatory dysfunction. While often considered, Colachis and Otis suggested this was an infrequent cause of fever.[5] Thus, of 713 febrile days, they found only 71 days (10%) of documented febrile episodes occurring, and 17 of 60 patients who were febrile could not be associated with established causes of fever. Careful search must be done for known causes of fever as previously noted before concluding thermoregulatory dysfunction is the cause of the fever.

|Lastly, other causes of fever to be considered include wound abscesses, particularly at the site of surgery or prior injury, and intra-abdominal inflammations or infections, such as cholecystitis, appendicitis, or diverticulitis. Of course, other causes of fever occurring in ambulatory patients must also be kept in mind.

References

1. Sugarman B, Brown D, Musher D. Fever and infection in spinal cord injury patients. *JAMA* 1982;248:66-76.

2. Beraldo PS, Neves EG, Alves CM, et al. Pyrexia in hospitalized spinal cord injury patients. *Paraplegia* 1993;31:86-191.

3. Colachis S, Otis S. Occurrence of fever associated with thermoregulatory dysfunction after acute traumatic spinal cord injury. *Am J Phys Rehab* 1995;74:114-119.

4. Wheeler JS, Walter JW. Acute urologic management of the patient with spinal cord injury. *Urologic Clinics of No Am* 1993;20:403-411.

5. Perkash I, Giroux J. Clean intermittent catheterization in spinal cord injury patients: a follow up study. *J Urology* 1993;149:1068-1071.

6. Chai T, Chung AK, Belville WD, Faeber GJ. Compliance and complications of clean intermittent catheterization in the spinal cord injured patient. *Paraplegia* 1995;33:161-163.

7. King RB, Carlson CE, Melvine J, et al. Clean and sterile intermittent catheterization methods in hospitalized patients with spinal cord injury. *Arch Phys Med Rehab* 1992;73:798-802.

8. Peterson JR, Roth EJ. Fever bacteriuria and pyuria in spinal cord injured patients with indwelling urethral catheters. *Arch Phys Med Rehab* 1989;70:839-841.

9. Fuhrer MJ, Garber SL, Rintala DH, et al. Pressure ulcers in community-resident persons with spinal cord injury: prevalence and risk factors. *Arch Phys Med Rehab* 1993;74:1172-1177.

10. Cheshire DJ. Respiratory management in acute traumatic tetraplegia. *Paraplegia* 1964; 1:252-261.

11. Bellamy R, Pitts F, Stauffer E. Respiratory complications in traumatic quadriplegia: analysis of 20 years experience. *J Neurosurgery* 1973;39:596-600.

12. Goetter WE, Stover SL, Kuhlemeier K, Fine PR. Respiratory complications following spinal cord injury: a prospective study. *Arch Phys Med Rehab* 1986;67:628.

13. Reines HD, Harris RC. Pulmonary complications of acute spinal cord injuries. *Neurosurgery* 1987;21:193-196.

14. Fishburn MJ, Marino RJ, Ditunno J. Atelectasis and pneumonia in acute spinal cord injury. *Arch Phys Med Rehab* 1990;71:197-200.

15. Van Hove E. Prevention of thrombophlebitis in spinal cord injury patients. *Paraplegia* 1978;16:332-335.

16. Watson N. Venous thrombosis and pulmonary embolism in spinal cord injury. *Paraplegia* 1968;6:113-121.

17. Weingarden DS, Weingarden SI, Belen J. Thromboembolic disease presenting as fever in spinal cord injury. *Arch Phys Med Rehab* 1987;68:176-177.

18. Venier LH, Ditunno J. Heterotopic ossification in the paraplegic patient. *Arch Phys Med Rehab* 1971;59:475-479.

19. Tow A, Kong K. Prolonged fever and heterotopic ossification in a C4 tetraplegic patient: case report. *Paraplegia* 1995;33:170-174.

20. Garland DE. A clinical perspective on common forms of acquired heterotopic ossification. *Clin Orthop* 1991; 263:13-29.

FEVER
| Robert A. Kaplan, MD

in Patients With SCI
CHAPTER TWENTY-THREE ▇▇▇▇▇▇

|Although thermoregulation is disordered as part of the autonomic dysfunction in patients with complete thoracic and cervical spinal cord injuries (SCIs), and unexplained "quadriplegia fever" is a well-described phenomenon in the weeks following a injury, in general, body temperature measurements have the same clinical significance in patients with SCI as in the general population. A wide variety of infectious and non-infectious diseases may produce fever. This chapter will focus on those conditions that are especially common or problematic in patients with SCI and will present an approach to diagnosis and management.

|Among the common non-infectious causes of fever in patients with SCI are drug fevers, superficial or deep venous thrombophlebitis and pulmonary embolism, atelectasis, trauma, heterotopic ossification, pancreatitis, exposure to excessive ambient temperatures, and possibly the cord injury itself. Less common non-infectious causes include malignancies and collagen-vascular diseases. The most common infectious cause of fever is pyelonephritis due to neurogenic bladder and instrumentation. Other common infectious causes include pneumonia (especially, but not exclusively, in patients with cervical levels of injury), infected pressure sores with or without osteomyelitis, sinusitis (especially in the patient with nasogastric or nasotracheal intubation), cholecystitis, diverticulitis, other ruptured viscera, cystitis, prostatitis, epididymitis, and intravascular catheter and orthopedic hardware-related infections. Special groups of patients may be at risk for a broader variety of infections. For example, a patient who was recently hospitalized for antibiotic treatment for an infected wound may have fever and diarrhea due to *Clostridium difficile* colitis. A traveler to Africa may return with malaria. An intravenous drug abuser may have primary HIV infection or AIDS with an opportunistic infection or malignancy.

|A thorough history and physical examination are essential in the evaluation of the febrile patient with SCI, both to elucidate distinctive epidemiologic features and to target the likely site of disease. Features of particular importance in the history include the timing, level, and completeness of the cord injury, any associated injuries, antecedent medical conditions, drug allergies, and the details of the post-injury course (hospitalizations, drug therapy including antibiotics, prior infections, procedures, complications, and instrumentation). Distinguishing symptoms of the febrile illness may be obscured by sensory deficits, but careful questioning may yield important localizing clues and guide further investigation. Skin changes, increased spasticity, headache, dyspnea, lightheadedness, diaphoresis, nausea, and a change in the appearance, amount, or odor of urine may be the only indicators of infection below the level of injury. Classic pain patterns and radiation may be altered, with focal pain more likely to be present above the level of injury.

|On physical examination, special attention should be paid to the patient's general appearance. Facial expression, respiratory pattern, coloration, and body position may be indicators of the severity of disease. Acute hypertension suggests autonomic dysreflexia, with fever potentially due to infection related to a distended viscus. Hypotension may be a sign of sepsis. Examination of the entire skin surface must be performed to search for ulcers and inflammatory changes, especially at intravenous catheter sites and pressure points. Sinus tenderness should be elicited. Chest examination may find evidence of consolidation, atelectasis, or effusion. A pathologic murmur may be a clue to endocarditis.

|The abdominal examination is often clouded by the neurologic deficits. Tenderness, guarding, and rebound tenderness may be absent even in the presence of peritonitis. Occasionally, increased spasticity of the abdominal musculature overlying an inflammatory process may be noted. Rectal and genital examinations may also suggest inflammation. The extremities should be examined for asymmetric edema indicating possible deep venous thrombosis.

|Laboratory and imaging evaluation is best guided by the history and physical examination. A complete blood count with differential and a urinalysis with microscopic examination are routine. Blood cultures, Gram stains, and cultures of urine, sputum, and other potentially infected material are usually necessary to establish the bacteriologic diagnosis. Note that bacteriuria is very prevalent in the healthy SCI population; pyuria and systemic signs of infection should be sought to establish the urinary tract as the source of fever. Furthermore, polymicrobial bacteriuria is common. Chest and abdominal films and serum chemistries (including electrolytes, blood urea nitrogen and creatinine, liver chemistries, amylase, and lipase) are often helpful. The erythrocyte sedimentation rate, although generally not providing specific diagnostic information, may be a useful gauge in following the response to therapy. If osteomyelitis is suspected, careful correlation of bone films, bone scanning, and gallium scanning will usually separate bone from soft-tissue inflammation as a prelude to bone biopsy and culture; indium-labeled white cell scanning, CT, and MRI may provide additional information. If intra-abdominal pathology is suspected, ultrasonography and CT scanning are useful; abdominal fluid collections can often be drained percutaneously for diagnosis. Only rarely is a diagnostic laparotomy or laparoscopy indicated without some clue from physical examination, laboratory results, or imaging. If urinary tract pathology is suspected, renal ultrasound (and under certain circumstances intravenous or retrograde urography) is indicated to look for hydronephrosis, stones, or other anatomical lesions. If pulmonary embolism is suspected, arterial blood gas measurement and electrocardiography may suggest the diagnosis, but ventilation/perfusion scanning or spiral CT (and occasionally pulmonary angiography) are necessary to substantiate the diagnosis and provide support for a decision to begin long-term anticoagulation. If deep venous thrombosis is suspected, then venous Doppler ultrasound or venogram is indicated.

|Management of the febrile patient with SCI must obviously be individualized and must take into account available resources and prevailing institutional antibiotic susceptibility patterns. The intensity of diagnostic evaluation and the rapidity with which therapy is instituted depend on the severity of the febrile illness; no algorithm can substitute for good clinical judgement. The well-appearing patient with low-grade fever may be followed expectantly whereas the hypotensive patient with rigors may need fluid and pressor support, immediate administration of parenteral broad-spectrum antibiotics, and urgent surgical and/or urologic evaluation. Among the common etiologies of fever in the patients with SCI, bacterial sepsis (especially related to infection behind obstruction or to a perforated viscus) and pulmonary embolism can be the most rapidly catastrophic. In the severely ill febrile patient with SCI, consideration of these diagnoses should prompt an urgent diagnostic evaluation with institution of empiric therapy as the evaluation proceeds.

|Some generalizations can be made about antibiotic therapy in the patient with SCI. Vascular, urinary tract, and respiratory tract instrumentation, long hospitalizations, and frequent antibiotic use are associated with frequent colonization and infection with resistant nosocomial pathogens, such as methicillin-resistant *Staphylococcus aureus* and a variety of Gram-negative bacilli. Commonly used antibiotic combinations, such as ampicillin and gentamicin, may be inactive against infections with these organisms. Empiric antibiotics should be chosen based on local sensitivity patterns. In the SCI unit at our institution, empiric therapy for urinary tract infections usually consists of an antipseudomonal penicillin and amikacin. Vancomycin is often included in regimens for skin and soft-tissue infection. (See chapter 18 on decubitus ulcers.)

|Altered volume of distribution and elimination kinetics may produce unpredictable serum antibiotic levels in patients with SCI. Antibiotics with narrow therapeutic indices, such as aminoglycosides, require careful drug level monitoring to help ensure efficacy and avoid toxicity.

|Although rationally chosen antibiotics, adjusted based on culture results, are necessary for adequate therapy of bacterial infections in patients with SCI, antibiotics alone are inadequate for treatment of abscesses, infection behind obstruction, infected kidney stones, ruptured viscera, and chronic osteomyelitis. In these settings, surgical or radiologic intervention is indicated.

|When unexplained fever persists despite an extensive evaluation, occult or exotic infection, collagen-vascular disease, or malignancy may be present. Infectious disease consultation may be helpful to guide further work-up. (See chapters 21 and 22 on thermoregulation and infections in SCI.)

Suggested Reading

I. Darouiche RO, Musher DM. Infections in patients with spinal cord injury. In: Mandell GL, Bennett JE, Dolin R, (Eds). *Principles and Practice of Infectious Diseases, Fourth Edition*. Churchill Livingstone: New York, 1995; pp. 2732-2737.

II. Schmidt KD, Chan CW. Thermoregulation and fever in normal persons and in those with spinal cord injury. *Mayo Clinic Proceedings* 1992;67(5)69:469-475.

|PSYCHIATRIC

James N. Nelson, MD

Emergencies in Patients With SCI

CHAPTER TWENTY-FOUR ▆▆▆▆▆▆▆▆▆▆

|An injury to the spinal cord or central nervous system requires early intervention and intensive follow-up to reduce the physical disability as much as possible. This is also true of the trauma to the psychological well-being of the patient. Early involvement and intensive follow-up by the mental health team can make a difference in the psychological adjustment and overall attitude of the patient with a spinal cord injury (SCI).[1] Evidence of the psychological impact is clear with the suicide rate among individuals with SCI five times higher than in the general population.[2]

|It is important that the inevitable depression and psychological adjustment problems be given early attention. It is of interest that in the patient with SCI, the suicide rate is higher for women, and the suicide rate for the less disabled is twice as high as the severely disabled. A significant partner relationship and good family support has a profound impact on depressive feelings and perception of a good quality of life in patients with SCI.[3] Of course, the psychological status of the patient prior to the SCI is significant in the long-term adjustment. It is important that how the patient thinks and feels is not ignored. Recovery from SCI requires considerable problem-solving and coping strategies by the patient. It appears that patients with SCI with a family history of alcoholism use different coping methods and behaviors. This finding suggests different therapeutic approaches for these groups.[4] Consultation with, and being a part of, a drug and rehabilitation program is a valuable part of the psychological evaluation and follow-up of the patient with SCI.

|At any point in the care of the patient with SCI, a psychiatric crisis can occur. A sudden mental status change qualifies as a psychiatric emergency because intrusive suicidal thoughts can occur without warning. Agitation, confusion, and disorientation can be a part of an infection, temperature elevation, and a physical problem, or it can be signs of withdrawal from chronic overuse of barbiturates, alcohol, bromoseltzer, or other drug that produces withdrawal symptoms. Admission to the hospital—from the initial injury to any subsequent admission— can result in withdrawal symptoms.

|The higher suicide risk has been mentioned and any signs or symptoms that suggest thoughts of suicide should be taken seriously and acted on immediately. Any concerns by any team member should be shared and the psychiatric team called. A matter-of-fact discussion with patient and the treatment team, with a plan that can include one-to-one observation, can be comforting to the patient and the staff.

|The patient with SCI can have any unexpected reaction to medication. Segal and Brunneman point out that absorption of oral or IM medication can be very different in patients with SCI.[5] They are at increased risk for anticholinergic delirium from diphenhydramine and tricyclic antidepressants.

|The neuroleptic malignant syndrome in patients on psychotropic medication is a psychiatric emergency. Fever or confusion should prompt an evaluation for neuroleptic malignant syndrome, which includes muscle rigidity and autonomic instability. All antipsychotic medications should be discontinued. Supportive treatment and use of the dopamine agonist bromocriptine, from 2.5 mg BID up to 15 mg daily, can be life saving. The earlier the diagnosis, the easier the course of treatment.

|Sudden withdrawal from baclofen can produce psychotic symptoms. Low doses of haloperidol or risperidone can relieve the hallucinations and disorganized thinking until baclofen can be resumed.

|SCI can accentuate personality defects. A psychiatric emergency can result from verbally and physically abusive patients. The patient can split the treatment team by being cooperative with certain staff members and uncooperative with others. Psychiatric intervention may be necessary in these situations. A diagnostic formulation and a treatment plan, to which all members of the treatment team contribute, is the beginning of any help for the patient. In an emergency, one can give haloperidol 2 mg, lorazepam 2 mg, and benztropine 2 mg IM to calm an agitated patient.

References

1. Craig, Hancock, and Dickson. Improving the long-term adjustment of spinal cord injured patients. *Spinal Cord* 1999;37(5):345-350.

2. Hartkopp, Bronnum-Hansen,Seidenschnur, Biering-Sorensen. Suicide in a spinal cord injured population. *Arch Phys Med and Rehab* 1998;79(11):1356-1361.

3. Kreuter, Sullivan, Dahllof, and Siosteen. Partner relationships, functioning, mood and global quality of life in persons with spinal cord injury and traumatic brain injury. *Spinal Cord* 1998;36(4):252-261.

4. Schandler, Cohen, Vulpe. Problem solving and coping strategies in persons with spinal cord injury who have and do not have a family history of alcoholism. *J of Spinal Cord Medicine*, 1996;19(2):78-86.

5. Segal JL, Brunneman SR. Clinical pharmacokinetics in patients with spinal cord injury. *Clinical Pharmacokinetics* 1989;17(2):109-129.

NURSING
Cathy Parsa, BSN, MA, CRRN; Anita Cordova, MSN, CRRN

Management of the Complications of SCI
CHAPTER TWENTY-FIVE ▰▰▰▰▰▰▰▰▰▰▰▰

The following information is provided as an overview for nurses working with persons with spinal cord injury (SCI) in acute medical, rehabilitation, and community settings. The promotion of wellness and prevention of life-threatening complications are major nursing responsibilities. SCI nursing is a unique specialty and the nurse must be knowledgeable about the numerous ways in which an injury affects the person and the various body systems. This knowledge base, along with technical skills, sound clinical judgment, and well-developed interpersonal skills, will make prevention and/or timely assessment of complications possible.

The level and completeness of the person's injury gives the nurse a clue to the changes in body functions and potential complications the patient may experience. However, keep in mind that every SCI is different and biopsychosocial make-up of each person will influence his or her response to the injury as well as the interventions. Also remember to consider how pre-existing conditions and the aging process affect the type and severity of complications.

|For a more comprehensive discussion of this topic we highly recommend *Management of Spinal Cord Injury* (Second Edition), edited by Cynthia Perry Zejdlik.[1] Also, the Consortium for Spinal Cord Medicine, supported by the Paralyzed Veterans of America, has developed a series of clinical practice guidelines that are important resources for any health care professional in the field.[2]

Complications of the Respiratory System

|The level of SCI will determine the neurological control of breathing and anticipated dysfunction. The muscles of breathing, cough function, and vital capacity are important considerations in maintaining optimal respiratory function. Persons with injuries located above T10 experience changes in the function of key muscles involved in respiration and are at increased risk of complications. Decreased vital capacity, ineffective cough, and changes in mobility lead to an increased tendency toward atelectasis and pneumonia.

|Ensure adequate hydration to keep secretions viscous and use the assisted or quad cough technique as needed to help keep lungs clear. Percussion and postural drainage, as well as suctioning during periods of respiratory infection may be advised. Encourage increased mobility, coughing and deep breathing exercises, and the use of an elastic abdominal binder to support the diaphragm when up in the wheelchair. The respiratory therapist should be consulted for exercises to increase vital capacity. Of course cessation of smoking is critical to promote healthy lung function.

|Hypoxia and sleep apnea are usually related to impaired neural impulses or low cardiac output. Restlessness or irritability is an early sign of hypoxia; other signs may include rapid, shallow breathing, dyspnea, and pallor. If a problem is suspected, oxygen saturation should be monitored; oxygen therapy is the typical treatment.

|A tracheostomy tube may be placed to assist with short- or long-term maintenance of bronchial hygiene and ease of respiratory effort. Persons with complete injuries above C4 typically require permanent respiratory support. Portable ventilators are frequently used and have proved to be very reliable. Back-up systems must be kept available along with a manual resuscitation (ambu) bag and suction equipment.

|The existence of a tracheostomy tube (with or without mechanical ventilation) increases the risk of infection. Thick secretions or mucous plugs in the artificial airway can cause obstruction. Tracheoesophageal fistula can result from necrosis of the posterior wall of the trachea. Scarring may lead to stenosis and granulation that can cause tracheal obstruction. Infections can occur at the stomal site and communication problems must be addressed. (See chapter 4 on respiratory emergencies.)

|Pulmonary emboli (PE), another complication, usually arise from a deep venous thrombosis (DVT) in the lower extremities. Decreased mobility, cardiovascular changes, surgery, and soft-tissue damage can all lead to an increased risk. Low-grade fever, shortness of breath, chest pain, and blood-tinged sputum may be observed. Small emboli may go undetected while a large one may lead to a respiratory arrest. The lung scan has proven to be a reliable, non-invasive diagnostic tool. Anticoagulation therapy is administered to prevent further embolization. (See chapter 10 on DVT.)

Complications of the Cardiovascular System

|Some persons with cervical cord injury are especially prone to cardiac dysrhythmias. Stimulation, such as suctioning or rapid changes in body position, may lead to an abnormal vasovagal response, which can cause uncontrolled bradycardia or cardiac arrest. Observe for changes in level of consciousness, falling blood pressure and pulse, irregular pulse, decreased urinary output, dependent edema, and/or pulmonary edema. Maintain normal fluid and electrolyte balance, monitor laboratory results and administer medications and oxygen as ordered. (See chapter 2 on cardiovascular system.)

|Circulatory return to the heart is poor and, along with loss of muscle mass, may lead to dependent edema. Encourage mobility and ensure that lower extremities are supported with leg extenders while the person is in a wheelchair and with pillows when in bed. Use elastic stockings as necessary.

|In SCI, baseline blood pressure is low and sluggish circulation contributes to a dramatic fall in blood pressure when the person is placed in an upright position (known as postural or orthostatic hypotension). Elastic stockings and/or an abdominal binder may help. Also encourage a slow rise to sitting position. Signs and symptoms are typically dizziness and blurred vision. Fainting may occur. Management involves lowering the person's head and occasionally administering medication to boost blood pressure. Over time, compensatory mechanisms decrease problems in this area.

|Autonomic dysreflexia, also known as hyperreflexia, is a potentially fatal complication that occurs in injuries above the T6 level. The rapid and significant elevation (systolic over 150 mmHg or 20 to 40 mmHg above baseline) of blood pressure is the concern here.

|The cause can be any irritating or noxious stimuli with bladder overdistention being the most common problem. Signs and symptoms include one or more of the following: pounding headache, profuse sweating above the level of injury, goose bumps, flushing, blurred vision, nasal congestion, feelings of anxiety, and cardiac arrhythmias.

|First-line treatment for autonomic dysreflexia involves placing the person in a sitting position (in order to lower blood pressure) and obtaining a blood pressure reading. Assess for potential causes (again, bladder distention is the most common) and take corrective action. Pharmacologic management may be necessary, especially if the blood pressure remains elevated above 150 mmHg. Antihypertensives with rapid onset and short duration are most useful, but may cause hypotension. Continue to monitor the individual for at least two hours after resolution of the episode. Refer to the clinical practice guidelines, "Acute Management of Autonomic Dysreflexia," from the Consortium for Spinal Cord Medicine for a complete, step-by-step protocol. (See chapter 1 on autonomic dysreflexia.)

|DVT is common in lower extremities in patients with acute SCI with a somewhat lower risk in patients with chronic injuries. Decreased mobility, cardiovascular changes, surgery, and soft-tissue damage increase risk. Smoking should be discouraged due to its effects on the circulatory system. Use correct positioning to decrease pressure on major blood vessels, and avoid lower extremity venous puncture. Signs and symptoms include an increase in calf or thigh circumference, pain or tenderness, localized redness or warmth, and low-grade fever. Note that some persons will be asymptomatic. Doppler ultrasound, 125-I fibrinogen scanning, and contrast venography can be used to confirm a diagnosis.

|Aggressive medical prophylaxis for acute injuries is necessary and mechanical (compression hose, pneumatic devices, and vena cava filter placement) as well as anticoagulant interventions are recommended. In chronic SCI, prophylactic measures should be considered during periods of prolonged bed rest or following surgical procedures. Additionally, DVT may be a cause of autonomic dysreflexia.

Complications of the Integumentary System

|Skin is the body's largest organ and plays a vital role in maintaining health. Changes in circulation, mobility, and sensation after SCI increase susceptibility to breaks in skin integrity. In turn, this can lead to increased length of stay or rehospitalization, increased cost of care, surgery, loss of limb, and, in the most severe cases, loss of life. Pressure, shearing, and trauma are the primary causes of problems. Use of pressure-relieving equipment (mattresses and cushions), correct positioning and posture, regular position changes, adequate nutrition and hydration, and good personal hygiene are the basic prevention techniques. Skin breakdown is often more highly correlated to attitude and psychosocial factors than to level of injury and functional ability. Regularly scheduled skin inspections lead to early detection of problems and, consequently, less severe breakdown.

|Skin breakdown is an all-inclusive term. Pressure sores or ulcers refer to damage caused by excessive pressure. A four-step staging system is commonly used to classify pressure sores and management is based on classification as well as resources available and the preferences of the health care team or individual. In all cases, the cause of the pressure sore needs to be identified and removed. Devitalized tissue needs to be removed and the wound bed kept moist (but not wet) and clean to promote healing. Continual evaluation of the effectiveness of interventions is vital. An enterostomal (ET) nurse is a valuable resource to the health care team.

|Be aware that skin is more susceptible to breakdown when edema is present and during febrile states. Skin care routines may need to be stepped up at those times. Aging skin is drier and less resilient so patients who have no history of skin problems may begin to experience them in later stages of life. Ingrown toenails and resultant localized infections are another common complication. (Toenails should be cut straight across and not too short.) Any type of skin breakdown may become a potential cause of autonomic dysreflexia and also cause an increase in spasms.

Complications of the Genitourinary System

|Neurogenic bladder and sphincter are an expected result of SCI secondary to the disruption of nerve pathways. The kidneys and production of urine are unaffected but problems occur with storage and voiding. The exact nature of dysfunction can be determined by urodynamic study. The results, along with consideration of the person's preferences, lifestyle, resources, and abilities lead to selection of an appropriate bladder management program. Typically one or more of the following interventions are used: intermittent catheterization, indwelling urethral or suprapubic catheters, external (condom) catheters, trigger or reflex voiding. Medications to reduce bladder spasms or decrease sphincter tone may also be used and a sphincterotomy may be performed. The goal of every program is to provide complete and predictable emptying to decrease the risk of urinary tract infection (UTI) and prevent high bladder pressures that may lead to reflux and kidney damage. (See chapter 7 on urology emergencies.)

|The incidence of UTI in the SCI population is high and most persons have bacteria in their urine most of the time. Treatment is typically reserved for those who become symptomatic (increased temperature, general malaise, cloudy and foul-smelling urine, and leakage around the catheter). Prevention focuses on regular emptying, maintenance of clean or sterile technique, and adequate fluid intake. Autonomic dysreflexia and an increase in spasms may be seen. Monitor labs (urine analysis and culture and sensitivity are commonly performed) and administer antibiotics and antipyretics as ordered.

|UTI, metabolic imbalance, decreased mobility, and the presence of a foreign body (catheter) all contribute to the formation of urinary calculi or renal stones. The risk is minimized with an effort to reduce UTIs, maintaining acidic urine (by increasing administration of ascorbic acid), and encouraging mobility and hydration. Small stones may pass, but larger ones can cause an obstruction. It is vital to monitor urinary output on a regular basis. Stones may be removed by transurethral crushing or shockwave lithotripsy. Urease inhibitors and bladder irrigation may also be prescribed. In males, be aware of the complications of acute epididymitis and be aware of the presence of penile implants and any complications related to them.

Complications of the Gastrointestinal System

|Neurogenic bowel and sphincter are also expected after an SCI. Dysfunction is typically determined by the location and completeness of the injury and is highly associated with patterns of bladder dysfunction. Motility is generally sluggish (accentuated with aging) and the sensation and ability to defecate are affected. A regular bowel program must be established and maintained and takes into consideration the type of dysfunction, past bowel habits, functional abilities, personal preferences, and resources available. The goal is to establish a pattern of predictable and complete emptying. Adequate fluid intake, a balanced diet, ingestion of high-fiber foods, and an active lifestyle are important components of an effective program.

|Medications, such as bulk-forming laxatives, stool softeners, suppositories, and stimulant laxatives, may have a place in the bowel program, but should not be overused. Enemas should generally be avoided as they contribute to loss of bowel tone over time. Constipation is one of the more common complications and may progress to impaction. Monitor for signs and symptoms that include loss of appetite, abdominal distention or discomfort, nausea or vomiting, and oozing of liquid or loose stool. An abdominal X-ray can confirm the diagnosis. Treatment will require vigorous intervention including strong cathartics. Note that after a complete clean-out, it is necessary to wait a few days before restarting the bowel program.

|Diarrhea usually results from the ingestion of new foods, alcohol, excessive use of laxatives, new medication, stress, or anxiety. Replace fluids and electrolytes and keep the skin clean. If the diarrhea lasts more than three days, consider whether it may be part of an infective process. Observe for an increase in temperature and a change in the color and/or odor of the stool. Have a specimen analyzed if necessary.

|Manual (digital) stimulation of the rectum (a commonly used technique), long periods of time on the commode chair, and straining all contribute to the formation of hemorrhoids. These may occur outside the anal sphincter (where they are visible) or internally. They may bleed and become infected; they may also cause autonomic dysreflexia, as can other problems related to the gastrointestinal system or bowel program.

|Colostomies are performed in cases of rectal prolapse or to prevent fecal contamination of pressure sores in the perineal area. They may also be considered in individuals who have extreme difficulty with evacuation due to megacolon and have exhausted all other avenues. The Consortium for Spinal Medicine recommends that colorectal cancer be ruled out in patients with SCI over the age of 50 with a positive fecal occult blood test or a change in bowel function that doesn't respond to corrective actions.

Complications of the Musculoskeletal System

|Persons with an acute injury may still be healing a vertebral fracture. Depending on the type and location of the injury, they may have been surgically stabilized or use an orthotic device. Obtain clear instructions on activity allowed and maintenance of equipment. A halo vest will require regular pin care and assessment of skin under the vest. The nurse must also know how to remove the vest in case of emergency (need for CPR).

|Heterotopic ossification (HO) is the formation of new bone around joints and can cause severe pain (a potential cause of autonomic dysreflexia and increased spasms) and immobility. Additional signs and symptoms include localized redness and swelling, local and systemic temperature elevation, and stiffness (note some similarities to DVT). Bone scanning and X-ray may be used to confirm diagnosis. Treatment consists of range of motion associated with exercises, increased activity, medication, radiation, and, in extreme cases, surgical removal of the abnormal bone formation.

|Pathological fractures of the long bones are common due to porosity and softness related to immobility and incidence also increases with age. Minor trauma can cause a fracture. Assess for localized swelling and redness, abnormal alignment, crepitus, and pain in persons with intact sensation. (See chapter 15 on fractures.)

|The presence of spasticity is primarily determined by the location and extent of the SCI. A small amount of spasticity is considered useful in maintaining circulation and muscle tone, prevention of DVT, and can even be used in functional activities such as transfers. On the other hand, too much spasticity can be uncomfortable, cause skin breakdown, increase the risk of falls, and contribute to the formation of contractures. A relatively sudden increase in the intensity of spasms may signal the existence of a DVT, PE, skin breakdown, infection, impaction, HO, fracture, etc.

|Management of spasticity includes proper positioning, range of motion exercises on a regular basis, epidural electrical stimulation, and medication. In severe cases, implanted intrathecal drug delivery systems (Baclofen pump), nerve blocks, and ablative surgical techniques may be used.

|Syringomyelia, cystic degeneration of the spinal cord at the site of the injury may cause pain (another potential cause of autonomic dysreflexia and increased spasticity) and progressive damage resulting in increased neurological deficit. Be alert to loss or change of sensation or function or a change in sweating patterns. Diagnosis is confirmed with MRI; options for treatment are limited but may include shunting or other surgery.

Disturbances in Temperature Regulation

|Changes in the sympathetic nervous system lead to a decreased ability to maintain a steady internal temperature. Patients with SCI tend to be poikilothermic, that is, they assume the temperature of their environment. This can cause serious problems, such as heat exhaustion or stroke, especially because their ability to sweat below the level of injury is typically impaired. Hypothermia may also be experienced as a result of vasomotor tone changes that cause a continuous loss of body heat. Know the patient's baseline temperature so you may determine if a particular reading is significant.

Psychosocial Considerations

|Depression is not uncommon in the SCI population and may be exacerbated by physical changes related to the aging process as well as loss of significant others and support systems over time. Also, some medications may increase feelings of depression. Suicide is a significant cause of death in the disabled population. Pre-morbid use of drugs and/or alcohol, perhaps a causative factor related to the injury itself, may continue to be a problem.

|Violence, another common cause of SCI in some parts of the country, may continue to be part of a person's environment and put him or her at risk for further harm. Emotional and/or physical abuse at the hands of a care provider is a currently unexplored area. It is safe to assume that many persons with an SCI, especially those who are dependent on others for physical care, are at risk for becoming victims. Some signs and symptoms of abuse include unexplained cuts, bruises, and fractures; poor hygiene; anxiety; pressure sores; increased hospitalizations; etc.

Pain Syndromes

|Persons with acute and chronic SCIs commonly experience some type of pain. It is important to perform a complete work-up and eliminate pathological causes, such as syrinx, rotator cuff tears, and carpal tunnel syndrome. Five pain syndromes have been described in SCI: mechanical, peripheral, visceral, central, and psychogenic. Any type of pain may cause autonomic dysreflexia.

|Mechanical pain, usually located around the level of injury is the result of soft-tissue damage (including overuse) or the non-union of a spinal fracture. This type of dull, aching pain is also seen with the overuse of certain muscle groups such as in the shoulders. It is usually seen treated with physical therapy modalities and analgesics.

|Peripheral nerve root pain arises from damage at the site of the injury. It is usually sharp, stabbing, or shooting in character. This type of pain is often difficult to treat. Physical therapy modalities and topical analgesics may help. A variety of surgical techniques have been tried with some success.

|Visceral pain originates in the abdominal organs, such as the bladder or bowel, and may be referred to the chest, shoulder or suprapubic areas.

|Central (or deafferentation) pain comes directly from the spinal cord and is the result of newly formed, non-functional nerve fiber growth. The pain is severe and can be experienced as burning, tingling, squeezing, and sharp, shooting, and stabbing. Segmental deafferentation pain is felt around the level of injury. Phantom deafferentation pain is perceived below the level of injury where sensory loss is assumed. Surgical treatment maybe considered when medications fail.

|Psychogenic pain may be considered when the other types have been ruled out. It should be noted that all types of pain have emotional, psychological, social, and cultural influences. All pain is real and should be taken seriously. In addition to analgesics, anticonvulsants, and antidepressants have been found useful in treating some types of pain. Heat/cold, biofeedback, functional electrical stimulation (FES), and other physical therapy modalities also have a place in pain management.

Conclusion

|SCI nursing requires specialized knowledge and skills that have only been briefly addressed in this chapter. Interventions directed at preventing complications and early detection of problems will lead to positive outcomes. Patients with SCI and their families must be included in all aspects of care and receive the information necessary for them to maintain wellness throughout their life.

Note: This chapter was based on work originally written by Marilyn Wullschleger, BSN, MA, RN (deceased).

References

1. *Management of Spinal Cord Injury, Second Edition*, Perry Zejdlik C. (ed). Jones and Bartlett Publishers: Boston, 1992.

2. Consortium for Spinal Cord Medicine Clinical Practice Guidelines: *Prevention of Thromboembolism in Spinal Cord Injury* (1997); *Neurogenic Bowel Management in Adults with Spinal Cord Injury* (1998); and *Acute Management of Autonomic Dysreflexia* (1998).

PSYCHOSOCIAL
Helen T. Bosshart, ACSW/LCSW

Emergencies for Patients With SCI
CHAPTER TWENTY-SIX ▰▰▰▰▰▰▰▰▰

The patient with spinal cord injury (SCI) faces tremendous challenges to ensure that health care and social needs are met in the community. In addition to the issues addressed by the able-bodied in every day life, the person with SCI often has disability-related needs. Acquiring and maintaining accessible housing, transportation, adaptive equipment, and personal care assistance can pose formidable challenges. In spite of the best planning and coordination, problems will inevitably occur. Events that might be an inconvenience for someone without a disability present a genuine psychosocial emergency for the person with SCI. If the psychosocial emergency is not addressed and resolved, it may lead to costly health complications. Some of the most frequently reported social problems and possible solutions will be addressed.

Personal Care Assistance

"My caregiver didn't show up today. I don't have anyone to get me up and do my bowel care."

"My personal care attendant quit this morning. He just walked out."

"My wife's mother is very ill and they have called the family to come. She needs to leave for California today and I don't know how long she will be gone. There isn't anyone else to take care of me."

"My mother learned today that she needs a total hip replacement. The surgery is scheduled next week and she won't be able to take care of me for at least six weeks after she gets out of the hospital."

|When the rehab center receives a phone call from a patient with one of the above problems, immediate action is required. Without adequate personal care assistance for a person who is dependent in activities of daily living, there can be life-threatening complications. Means and Bolton report that personal care assistance is one of the most frequently reported unmet needs for persons with SCI.[1] When the problem occurs, what do we do about it?

|In the case of a personal care assistant not showing up or quitting, it may be possible to arrange temporary support through a community home health agency if the person has insurance or some type of funding source. A local center for independent living (CIL) may be a resource for finding assistance as well. Getting the personal care assistant used by a friend to help out temporarily might also be an option. Every effort is made to resolve the crisis in the community and prevent the need for hospitalization. In extreme circumstances where there is no immediate solution, there may be no alternative other than hospitalization for psychosocial reasons until an acceptable plan can be developed to ensure the person's safety and appropriate care.

|In situations where there is adequate time for planning, it may be possible for the person with SCI to hire a personal care assistant to provide care in the home. Another possible solution is respite care if this service is available in the rehab center or some other community agency, e.g., assisted-living facility or community nursing home. Planned episodes of respite care on a regular basis may also be instrumental in preventing caregiver burnout and breakdown of the home support system.

|It is extremely important for the rehab center to provide patient/family education on personal care assistance management as an integral component of the rehabilitation program.[2] The importance of always having a back-up plan for care needs to be emphasized. Teaching good problem-solving skills to know how to manage in case of an emergency is also a crucial element of the rehab process.

Family Crisis

"My wife just walked out on me. She wants a divorce."

"My son was in a serious car accident."

"My daughter is pregnant and she's only 15."

|When a person with SCI calls a rehab team member to discuss a personal crisis, every effort is made to arrange appropriate counseling or referral to a community resource for support. The social worker, psychologist, chaplain, or rehab counselor can often provide the services needed.

Financial Crisis

"My social security check didn't come in the mail. It's a week past due. I can't pay any of my bills."

"My wife left me and she cleaned out my bank account. I don't even have enough money to buy groceries, let alone pay my bills."

|When this problem occurs, referrals to resources in the community can often provide some relief until income is re-established. The social worker may need to assist with letters or telephone calls to debtors to explain the circumstances and assist the person with SCI to maintain crucial services.

Housing

"I have everything I own in the U-Haul. I don't have anywhere to stay. Can I stay here tonight and you find me an apartment tomorrow?"

"My landlord just gave me an eviction notice. I have a week to find another place to live."

|When the person with SCI arrives at the medical center announcing the above predicaments, the social worker is usually consulted for assistance. Whereas with the ambulatory population a referral to the Salvation Army or other temporary lodging assistance program may be the usual course of action, most of these facilities are not wheelchair-accessible and equipped to meet the needs of a person with SCI. Giving the person with SCI information regarding wheelchair-accessible apartments/housing in the community is an appropriate course of action. Information regarding affordable hotels/motels in the interim is also appropriate. The person with SCI needs to assume responsibility for problem-solving and resolving this crisis, with guidance from the social worker or other staff as needed.

Abuse and Neglect

"I'm the home health nurse for Mr. B. His family is leaving him at home alone for lengthy periods of time. I don't think he's had a bath since I was there last week. He's losing weight and he has a bad sacral ulcer."

"I'm Mr. C's neighbor. It's really none of my business, but his wife has really gone off the deep end. She can't take care of herself, let alone him. Somebody needs to do something."

|Unfortunately, these are not uncommon case scenarios. When there is reason to suspect abuse or neglect, whether intentional or unintentional, immediate intervention is indicated. A referral to the Adult Protective Services Agency for investigation and evaluation is the appropriate course of action. If the person with SCI is in an unsafe environment, it may be possible to involve other family members for assistance to improve the level of care. Family counseling to resolve the current situation in the home may also be an option. In extreme situations, it may be necessary to proceed with alternative placement if the situation cannot be resolved. It is the ultimate responsibility of the Adult Protective Services Agency to investigate and take appropriate action.

Conclusion

|Living with SCI requires skills for addressing environmental and social needs, as well as health care needs. In spite of the quality of care provided in an inpatient rehabilitation program, the person with SCI cannot experience some of these situations until after discharge to the community. To best prepare the person with SCI to handle the myriad of real-life emergencies that are inevitable, it is incumbent upon the rehabilitation professionals to teach problem-solving skills as a part of the rehabilitation process. The person with SCI needs to feel equipped with the tools to manage a crisis, not be overwhelmed by it.

|It is also essential to provide the person with SCI information regarding community resources and to establish community linkages for support in times of crisis. The services offered through CILs can prove invaluable. Referrals to peer counseling or support groups may help establish relationships with individuals who have experienced and successfully resolved similar psychosocial problems.

|The person with SCI also needs to know that the resources at the SCI Center will always be available. Although it is important for the person with SCI to manage and direct his/her own life, just knowing that support and direction is available in times of distress may provide the security necessary to cope with the presenting crisis. Ensuring the person with SCI access to counseling, services, and the expertise of the rehabilitation staff as he/she leaves the rehab setting and ventures into community living should be a part of discharge preparation.

Table I **Psychosocial Emergencies**

Emergency Problem	Interventions
Personal care assistance	Train individual to hire/manage his own employee(s); home health agencies; independent living center; family members; Medicaid waiver programs; state funding options; referral to VA for veterans; community services programs.
Housing	Refer to emergency shelters if wheelchair accessible; referral/information on wheelchair-accessible apartments/housing, e.g., local realtor; assisted living; personal care homes; independent living center; nursing home placement.
Finances	Refer to community agencies for emergency assistance; Supplemental Security Income; Social Security Disability Insurance; VA for veterans who served during "war-time"; workman's compensation; Food Stamps; Aid to Families with Dependent Children.
Peer support/family support	Refer to independent living centers, local rehab hospitals; Paralyzed Veterans of America, National SCI Association.
Psychological distress/family crisis	Refer to mental health professional, e.g., social worker, psychologist, chaplain, rehab counselor, or psychiatrist.
Suspected abuse or neglect	Refer to Adult Protective Services Agency.
Transportation	Refer to local public transit authority, Area Agency on Aging, State Division of Rehabilitation Services, Medicaid taxi services, refer to VA for veterans, independent living centers, churches.
Home accessibility	Refer to independent living centers, civic groups, churches, State Division of Rehabilitation Services, refer to VA for veterans.
Vocational/ employment	Refer to state employment agency, independent living center, State Division of Rehabilitation Services, refer to VA for veterans.
Caregiver burnout	Refer to VA for respite for veterans, respite care through local hospitals/nursing homes, homemaker services through VA or state funding, local support groups, mental health professional, community services programs.

The National SCI Hotline, 800 526-3456 (800 638-1733 in Maryland) can be a referral resource for federal/state/local assistance as well.

References

1. Means BL, Bolton B. Recommendations for expanding employability services provided by independent living programs. *Journal of Rehabilitation* 1994;4:20-25.

2. DeGraff AH. *Home Health Aides: How to Manage the People Who Help YOU*. Saratoga Access Publications: Clifton Park, NY;1988.

A